Contents

Introduction

But why do we need to change?

Frightening fact: across the NHS we currently harm around 1 in 10 patients.

Most complaints from patients and relatives are due to human factors. The Medical Protection Society states that 80% of litigation is due to human factors. Most people on the frontline in healthcare have little or no idea of the meaning of the term 'human factors'.

The time has come to fill in the gaps. The time has come to promote safety-positive behavioural culture change.

There is now a realization that knowledge and competence are not enough, and without what are now termed 'non-technical skills', fatal errors can and do occur. I like to think of human factors as the metaphorical glue that surrounds knowledge and skills. It is also the link between the individual and the systems which govern how they work, the environment they find themselves in, the equipment with which they work, and the team or teams that they interact with, as well as interacting with the patient.

These 'soft skills' are perhaps perceived as not as exciting as wielding a scalpel and yet it is these same soft skills which are what holds a life-saving emergency procedure together.

The communication, the leadership and team working, the task management, the decision-making, the situational and risk awareness, the error management, and the systems approach to safety are essential skills worthy of a place in medical education.

As history unfolds, it seems often to be the case that it is only following a crisis that we gather sufficient inertia to set about initiating change. I hope that the Mid Staffordshire NHS Foundation Trust Public Inquiry (Francis Report) will be one such turning point in healthcare. I wish to help initiate the new ideal of a 'learning culture with continuous improvement'.

I hope by the end of the book you will want to join with me to produce this overdue change.

Limited pockets of enthusiasm

It is true to say that there are areas who have grasped the nettle firmly. For example, the anaesthetists and surgeons have developed ANTS and NOTSS (anaesthetic non-technical skills and non-technical for surgeons) and there is now a chapter in the ALS manual devoted to human factors. However, research indicates that the majority of healthcare workers have little or no understanding of the term or the skills, attitudes, and behaviours that underpin this discipline.

What to expect in the chapters ahead

A new model for human factors by healthcare professionals for healthcare professionals has been developed. The approach takes you through a step-by-step process to become more self-aware of your own human factors and how to improve them.

Human interaction, task management, team working, ergonomics, environmental and equipment design, and designing systems with safety in mind are explored in depth.

The topic of error is covered in a way that encourages the focus to be on successful error management rather than blame with a 'big stick' idealism. The method promotes a move towards a risk-aware culture where people are open and willing to learn from their mistakes.

Examples of poor behaviour are unfortunately far too common within the NHS environment. This behaviour has gone unchallenged for years and in some places has been accepted as the norm. The time has come to equip people with a new skill set that encourages this behaviour to be challenged (see Example 1).

Example 1 Examples of poor behaviour

As a junior doctor, I witnessed equipment being launched across an operating theatre in a sea of rage, regular humiliation of junior doctors and nursing staff, angry outbursts reducing staff to tears, patients being ignored, and people being just plain rude. I saw this behaviour go unchallenged, 'Oh, so and so, is always like that, it's just their way'.

A simple plan is suggested along with real examples to illustrate how best to employ tools to start to reverse this trend of acceptance of the status quo.

The true story that inspired the changes

In 2005, a mother of two young children died during the induction of anaesthesia (being put to sleep) for a routine operation. Her husband, an airline pilot with an interest in human factors, took the brave step of publicizing her story in order to promote human factors awareness in the healthcare setting.

If you are still unconvinced of the need for a fresh approach to training beyond skills and knowledge, then by watching the film that her husband has recorded perhaps you will be inspired to change your mind.[1] The transcript can be found at <http://www.chfg.org/resources/07_qrt04/Anonymous_Report_Verdict_and_Corrected_Timeline_Oct_07.pdf>.

Why move away from aeroplanes?

There are many parallels between high-reliability organizations (including the aviation and the nuclear industry) and healthcare but there are also many differences.

The central entity in healthcare is, of course, a patient, a human with their own human factors. There is an incomprehensible number of permutations of patient characteristics and however many types of aeroplanes there are, humans are more complex and as yet, not fully understood.

The cockpit of a plane is small and the size of the team is, therefore, far fewer. A theatre team is usually in the region of at least seven people. At a recent successful resuscitation following cardiac arrest locally, a retrospective count of the numbers of staff who were involved in the first hour revealed over 25 people. The logistics of coordinating a team of that size requires different skills.

The pilot goes down with his plane. Whilst that statement may sound callous, it is tinged with a large dose of realism. Were it to be suggested that the surgeon and anaesthetist be wired to a potassium infusion that would be triggered if the patient died, the cynic would suggest that rather fewer heroic, life-saving operations would be undertaken. Perhaps fewer of the more challenging operations would be performed in the more elderly or less healthy patients in whom we currently try even if there is only a small chance of success.

In healthcare, there are times when success cannot be guaranteed. I suspect that pilots may never have to utter, 'we gave it our best shot' or 'we threw everything we had at it'. In spite of increasing knowledge, skills, and equipment, there are huge holes in our understanding. There are times when no matter what is done, the battle is lost and patients die. There is no greater certainty in life than death. Not all planes will eventually crash. Pilots will not usually have to explain to a relative that their loved one has died.

Even within healthcare the range of differing skill sets is huge. The subspecialities in healthcare are extremely diverse. The psychiatrist needs a different type of communication skills from the emergency physician who needs a different skill set from the oncologist who in turn faces a different type of decision-making from the intensivist. The nurse running a busy clinic will have different organizational challenges from the sister in charge of a surgical ward who will allocate resources differently from the charge nurse on elderly care. The effective manager in rehabilitation will take a different approach to the one managing acute trauma admissions which will be different from dermatology clinic which requires differing thought processes when ensuring the coronary catheter lab is able to cope with care 24/7.

The staff and the systems are incredibly diverse and complex in healthcare. Whilst some of the underlying principles are generic and can be extracted from aviation, these principles do not go far enough. It is time to build on what can be learnt from other industries but then to immerse it fully into healthcare. The more subtle nuances are best understood by those within healthcare themselves.

It is time to climb off the proverbial soapbox and put 20 years of experience in healthcare to good use to share a human factors system adapted for healthcare by someone in healthcare.

Key points

- Human factors are responsible for the majority of litigation and complaints in healthcare.

- There needs to be a cultural shift to incorporate this new way of thinking.

- Knowledge and skills are just the basic tools and they are ineffective without an integrated human factors approach.

- We need to promote safety positive behaviour.

Reference

1. Carthey J, Clarke J. *Patient Safety First Campaign* (Safer Care Priority Programme). NHS Institute for Innovation and Improvement. Available at: <http://www.chfg.org/resources/07_qrt04/Anonymous_Report_Verdict_and_Corrected_Timeline_Oct_07.pdf>

1

Human factors: so what's it got to do with me?

Primum non nocere
First do no harm

Adapted from the Hippocratic Oath

Introduction

People are not perfect. We make mistakes. In fact, it is a certainty that both you and I will make a mistake at some point in the future. While I was training, a senior and very wise consultant colleague used to say to me, 'the further away you are from your last disaster, the closer you are to your next'.

A common attitude still exists, however, that mistakes are something that happen to someone else.

Another common misconception is that mistakes are made by 'bad' doctors or healthcare workers. Each of us is only human. Bad things do happen to good people. We need to move away from the ostrich approach to error.

Itiel Dror used an interesting analogy when speaking at a conference to encourage a new approach to error awareness. Imagine the security check at an airport. A person sits in front of an x-ray machine scanning bags. During that time, the individual has a choice of mental models. Imagine thoughts as a repeating message played in their head. If the message that is on repeat is, 'no bomb, no bomb, no bomb . . . '. How likely do you think it is that they will find a bomb when there is one? Now consider a different frame of reference, an assumption that every bag contains a bomb and you have to look for it, 'bomb, bomb, bomb . . . ' or 'Where's the bomb? Where's the bomb? Where's the bomb? . . . '

In healthcare we need a parallel question. We need to be looking for the next error. If we can anticipate the next potential error perhaps we can plan to put in extra layers of safety to try and prevent it. The concept of layers of safety brings me to James Reason.[1–3] Reason is the author of the Swiss cheese error model. Imagine a slice of Swiss cheese. It is full of holes. Imagine thin slices of cheese placed like slices of toast on a toast rack. If you move the slices of cheese backwards and forwards it is possible to line up all of the holes. Once all the holes are aligned it is possible to pass a knitting needle through the holes. The cheese represents the layers of safety. The knitting needle represents the error that slides through all the layers under certain conditions.

By adding more layers of cheese, surely it is possible to make every system safer? Unfortunately as more layers of safety are added, so a process becomes more complicated. As a process becomes more convoluted it takes longer. It is partly due to human nature, sometimes work load pressure and sometimes financial pressure that means if there is a quicker way to do something then this will be the route chosen. This leaves us in a dilemma: efficiency versus safety. How many layers of safety or checklists or protocols will people follow before they become disengaged and bypass procedures? We will expand on process mapping and safety systems in Chapter 3.

For now, I hope I've convinced you it will happen to you. No matter how good you are, no matter how careful you are, it could be your turn next. It could be my turn tomorrow. I hope to slightly alter your mind set to start looking for your next error.

Suppose now the unthinkable has happened.

You've made a mistake. Are you going to tell someone?

Have you ever made a mistake and not admitted to it? Should an error always be reported? Should you tell the patient? Does everyone? What about a near miss? How do you know if it's a serious error or not?

The definition of what constitutes a 'Never Event' has recently been more clearly defined. However, the terminology of a 'Serious Untoward Incident' (SUI) which has been replaced by Significant Event or Serious Incident Requiring Investigation (SIRI) or Serious Incident (SI) results in ambiguity. How to evaluate the degree of harm or potential harm varies both within and between institutions. In a specialism that promotes clear, unambiguous systems and a reduction in variation, there is a certain irony in this approach.

In one region local to me there have been 28 Never Events over 3 years and 1600 serious incidents requiring investigation in 1 year reported to the Strategic

Health Authority. This represents the tip of the iceberg with regard to overall events, those that were not reported, and the near misses. Learning from all these other events is currently lost. In addition, only some institutions make any attempt to do a 'memory check'. This is the process where the learning is revisited to ensure new groups can learn from old mistakes and that learning is not forgotten.

I hear a variety of excuses as to why people don't report a problem:

> 'I filled the form in last time and nothing happened. What's the point?'
> 'It takes too long to do the form. We were short staffed and it would have compromised patient care.'
> 'One of my friends got into trouble.'

Apathy, high workload, and the 'black hole phenomenon' all contribute adversely to sustaining a reporting culture. By the 'black hole' I refer to the sense of filling in a report with an expectation that 'someone' will do 'something'. The form is sent 'somewhere' and never heard of again. An investigation may or may not be triggered but the outcome is not shared. The learning does not take place at a local level, let alone across the organization and the loop is not closed. In discussion with those who receive the forms, the number of reports can be overwhelming. They feel they are a filter system to look at the serious end of the spectrum. Their expectations are that the person doing the reporting will initiate an action plan. My experience is that there is plenty of room for improvement in role and system clarity within reporting. The concept of learning from near misses and how we may go about that is a subject that needs further consideration.[4]

More worrying still are the institutions or departments where there are undercurrents of fear about the consequence of reporting. I have observed fear of reprisal, fear of disciplinary procedures, fear of job security, and fear of litigation. It is sad and disappointing that my experience when investigating this topic is that a 'blame culture' is alive and well in significant sections of the National Health Service (NHS).

There has been a push towards generating a 'no blame' culture. Unfortunately there are cases of malicious intent (e.g. Harold Shipman) where blame is appropriate. To establish whether this could be the case, the Incident Decision Tree is a useful tool (Figure 1.1).

The Institute for Health Improvement (IHI) and others have suggested using the term 'just culture'. For me, when we are encouraging the use of clean language, the word 'just' is too close to the word 'justice'. It has implications of blame enshrined within it. I prefer the terms 'open culture' and 'learning culture'. Culture change is a slow process but it is very necessary if we are serious about reducing errors and making safety a top priority.

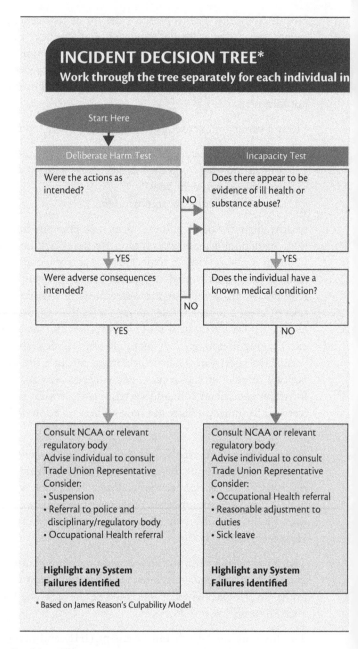

Figure 1.1 The Incident Decision Tree.
Reproduced from *The Incident Decision Tree: Information and advice on use*, National Patient Safety Agency, Figure 1, p. 3, Copyright © National Patient Safety Agency 2003. Licensed under the Open Government Licence v1.0. Source: Data from Reason J, *Managing the risks of organizational accidents*, pp. 191–222, Ashgate Publishing Group, Aldershot, UK, Copyright © 2003.

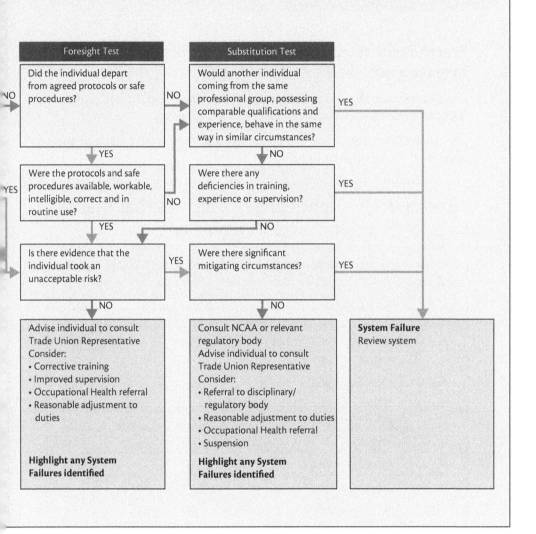

THE **NHS** CONFEDERATION

National Patient Safety Agency

Foresight Test	Substitution Test

Foresight Test

NO → Did the individual depart from agreed protocols or safe procedures? → NO

Substitution Test

Would another individual coming from the same professional group, possessing comparable qualifications and experience, behave in the same way in similar circumstances? → YES

↓ YES

↓ NO

YES → Were the protocols and safe procedures available, workable, intelligible, correct and in routine use? → NO

Were there any deficiencies in training, experience or supervision? → YES

↓ YES

↓ NO

Is there evidence that the individual took an unacceptable risk? → YES

Were there significant mitigating circumstances? → YES

↓ NO

↓ NO

Advise individual to consult Trade Union Representative
Consider:
• Corrective training
• Improved supervision
• Occupational Health referral
• Reasonable adjustment to duties

Highlight any System Failures identified

Consult NCAA or relevant regulatory body
Advise individual to consult Trade Union Representative
Consider:
• Referral to disciplinary/ regulatory body
• Reasonable adjustment to duties
• Occupational Health referral
• Suspension

Highlight any System Failures identified

System Failure
Review system

In times of financial cuts it is often assumed that cuts mean a compromise in quality. Wrong! By giving the right procedure/treatment/care, to the right patient, at the right time, in the right place, with the right equipment and the right staff with the right behaviours, right knowledge, and right skills we can prevent harm. By reducing harm we can save money.

The first step is increased error awareness.

Ever thought about when you are more likely to make a mistake?

If you have time, grab a pen and paper and try the following exercise (Exercise 1.1 'Identifying risk factors that make mistakes more likely').

If you don't have time or you don't learn like that, then at least take a moment to consider the question in Exercise 1.1.

Exercise 1.1 Identifying risk factors that make mistakes more likely

List the things you can think of that would increase the likelihood of you making a mistake. Count how many you have written before moving on.

So, if this was a Cosmo article (other women's magazines are available), I would now be giving you a graded rating scale in Table 1.1, telling you that if you identified over 150, then you can consider yourself very risk aware . . .

Table 1.1 Outward graded rating scale

<5	Less than average
5–10	Average
10–20	More than average
20–50	Well above average
50–250	Have you read the book before? (Tongue firmly in cheek!)

Our research has identified over 250 different contributors which make errors more likely and interfere with efficiency in the healthcare setting.

By raising your self awareness of the factors that make mistakes more likely, it is possible to tackle the next step and introduce systems to try to make it safer.

There are systems to be introduced at an organizational level but also personal behaviours that can become routine which can also alter outcomes. A random list of over 200 items is not terribly helpful. By developing a model it has been possible to link the items and identify common themes. Try Exercise 1.2 ('Factors in your last error or bad day').

Exercise 1.2 Factors in your last error or bad day

◆ Think back to your last bad day or the last error you witnessed.

◆ If you are struggling to imagine a bad day (you are one of the lucky ones!) then perhaps consider a poorly run critical incident or simply a series of events that resulted in inefficiency at some point from your past.

◆ List all of the things that contributed to the mistake or the inefficiency.

◆ Count the items and write down the number to come back to it later.

I want you to contrast the bad day with a good day. When things are going well—why is that? What makes it work well? What are the parallels that are present on both the good and the bad days?

If you are saying something broad like 'communication' or 'team work', start to ask yourself what does communication really mean to you? What makes it good? When does it go wrong? What is good team working? Why might you find it easier to work with one person than another?

What frustrates you? How efficient or objective do you remain once you are angry or overworked? How do you notice you are becoming stressed? What are your coping mechanisms?

What about the environment you work in? How easily can you find what you need? Do you ever get interrupted? How are the noise levels, lighting, and temperature?

Is the equipment you need always available in good working order? How well was it designed? Did the last person who used it clean it before they put it away or is there still blood on it?

Is there any order to your list, or is it random?

To move from random to ordered we have developed a new model. The SHEL model (Edwards 1972, International Civil Aviation Organization) and its derivative the SHELL model (Hawkins 1975), were developed in aviation. Attempts were made to adopt this model into healthcare[5] but it was found the aviation process models were not entirely applicable to healthcare settings. My colleagues and I therefore used grounded theory to produce a healthcare-focused model. This organic approach to change (i.e. developed by healthcare for healthcare) we felt would be more likely to embed effectively.

Introducing the new model

Did you notice what animal is on the front cover?

As I stood in front of my poster at a conference, I was asked if I came from Wales or New Zealand but the cover was inspired by the acronym I use for the new model: SHEEP as seen in Figure 1.2. The model appears in its entirety in Figure 1.3. Each of the five sections is considered in turn in more detail in the subsequent chapters.

The theory bit

For those of you who don't care how we developed the model you can skip the paragraph after Exercise 1.3. For the rest, a brief summary is included.

Exercise 1.3 Using the SHEEP sheet

◆ Think back to the situation that you considered in Exercise 1.2.

◆ Tick all the boxes on the 'SHEEP sheet' that were relevant.

◆ Compare how many items you identified in Exercise 1.2 using free recall, with how many ticks you have placed on the SHEEP sheet

S	ystems
H	uman interaction
E	nvironment
E	quipment
P	ersonal

Figure 1.2 The SHEEP model.

The study involved open questioning of over 250 human factors training course participants over 14 months drawn from all hospital staff (medical, nursing, and non-clinical—including a range of management/administrative/support staff). Open questions were used to gather data about what human factors influence staff efficiency and patient safety.

A grounded theory approach was used as the most appropriate method to develop a structured model of the relevant factors.[6] This enabled elicitation of an extensive range of as yet unknown factors and their relationships from varied participants.

After each training session of appropriately 12 participants the factors were analysed offline and structured into appropriate groups and duplicates removed. Axial coding involved investigating category relationships between the codes and established the primary groups based on accepted hospital norms.[7] This data was then used as a starting point for an iterative review, adjustment, and addition by follow-on groups through 20 cycles until no new factors were contributed (although courses and data capture and review continues). This process was similar to 20 PDSA cycles (Plan-Do-Study-Act) regularly used in the realm of health quality improvement. Other offline work included iterative elective coding of the most significant categories based on feedback, followed by identification of logically related concepts to optimize the form and ease of recognition of the model.

The SHEEP acronym was developed to enable easy memorization of the categories, whilst a metaphor was introduced, an allusion to the dangers of following blindly like sheep versus the imperative of the course to adopt 'safety positive' behaviours.

We have found that free recall resulted in an average of five to ten items being identified but by using the SHEEP sheet as an error checklist, it is possible to raise this number significantly.

Gawande[8,9] has convinced us of the usefulness of checklists rather then free recall in other settings. His amazing work has led to the introduction of the World Health Organization (WHO) theatre checklist which has been shown to have a positive impact on patient safety.[10]

I believe that in the setting of post 'error or near-miss' a checklist is invaluable in boosting the identification of contributory factors. If we don't identify the errors, how can we plan the learning that needs to follow? I would like you to consider the concept of the SHEEP detective who simply helps you look for clues.

On average the SHEEP sheet takes less than 10 minutes to complete.

In addition to using the SHEEP sheet as an error checklist retrospectively it can be used to help you become more risk aware. By producing a mental model

Systems

CULTURE

HOSPITAL CULTURE
- [ ] Departmental
- [ ] Professional
- [ ] Workgroup
- [ ] Mgmt vs. clinical
- [ ] Leadership culture

CULTURAL SYSTEMS LACK OF
- [ ] Open culture
- [ ] Safety culture
- [ ] Reporting Culture

INFORMATION FLOW CHOICE OF
- [ ] Face to face
- [ ] Phone
- [ ] Email
- [ ] Text
- [ ] Fax
- [ ] Access to info systems
- [ ] Access to info sets
- [ ] Breifing
- [ ] Debriefing
- [ ] Handover

INFORMATION SYSTEMS

MANUAL
- [ ] Patient notes
- [ ] Clinical pathway
- [ ] Care bundles

AUTOMATED APPLICATION
- [ ] Theatre mgmt
- [ ] Bed mgmt
- [ ] Pathology
- [ ] Patient mgmt

INFRASTRUCTURE
- [ ] Network
- [ ] Hardware

PRESCRIBED (SOP/Protocol/Guideline Issue)

- [ ] Failure to follow
  - [ ] *National*
  - [ ] *Local*
  - [ ] *Legal & Binding*
  - [ ] *WHO checklist*
  - [ ] *Care Bundle*
  - [ ] *Research*
  - [ ] *Professional Body*
- [ ] Lack of familiarity
- [ ] Different versions
- [ ] Ambiguity within
- [ ] Ambiguity between
- [ ] Unable to locate
- [ ] Chose to deviate due to
  - [ ] *Experience*
  - [ ] *Out of date*
  - [ ] *Inappropriate to situation*
- [ ] Refusal to use
- [ ] Complexity
- [ ] Not understood
- [ ] Conflicting rules/ guidelines

IMPROVEMENT MODELS LACK OF
- [ ] Productive ward
- [ ] TPOT (the productive operating theatre)
- [ ] Lean/6Sigma

ORGANIZATIONAL FLOW

PROBLEM WITH
- [ ] Clinical Department
- [ ] Business Department
- [ ] HR Department
- [ ] Finance Department
- [ ] IT Department
- [ ] Estates Department
- [ ] Quality Control
- [ ] Infection Control
- [ ] Security Systems

Personal

EXTERNAL INFLUENCES

PROBLEMS WITH
- [ ] Mood
- [ ] Frustration
- [ ] Emotional security
- [ ] Emotional trigger (events)
- [ ] Feeling unprepared
- [ ] Failure to achieve expectations
- [ ] Lack of self awareness
- [ ] Confidence
- [ ] Self esteem
- [ ] Motivation
- [ ] Lack of interest
- [ ] Complacency
- [ ] Denial of the situation
- [ ] Adaptability
- [ ] Ability to cope with major change
- [ ] Ability to cope with interruptions

PROBLEMS INFLUENCED BY WHO YOU ARE
- [ ] Race
- [ ] Gender
- [ ] Sexuality
- [ ] Personal value systems
- [ ] Personality (MBTI)
- [ ] Morals
- [ ] Cultural Identity

PATHOLOGY/PHYSIOLOGY
- [ ] Tired
- [ ] Hungry
- [ ] Thirsty
- [ ] Toilet break
- [ ] Health/illness
  - [ ] *Untreated (or)*
  - [ ] *On treatment*
- [ ] Stressed
- [ ] No energy
- [ ] Hormones/pregnancy

LIFE EVENTS
- [ ] Children
- [ ] Family
- [ ] Relationships
- [ ] Divorce
- [ ] Bereavement
- [ ] House move
- [ ] An argument
- [ ] Friends
- [ ] Commuting
- [ ] Parking
- [ ] Addiction to drugs
- [ ] Addiction to alcohol

ATTITUDES, BEHAVIOUR & EMOTION

MY WORK PROBLEMS WITH
- [ ] An argument
- [ ] Poor morale
- [ ] Time pressure
- [ ] Lack of planning time
- [ ] time
- [ ] Work time
- [ ] Rest time
- [ ] Work/rest balance
- [ ] Time of day
- [ ] Shift pattern
- [ ] Task conditions
  - [ ] *Elective*
  - [ ] *Scheduled*
  - [ ] *Urgent*
  - [ ] *Emergency*
  - [ ] *Clinical*
  - [ ] *Non clinical*
- [ ] High workload
- [ ] Lack of job satisfaction
- [ ] Job security
- [ ] Lack of team fit
- [ ] Lack of sense of belonging

Equipment

GENERIC PROBLEM WITH EQUIPMENT ITSELF

- [ ] Fitness for task
- [ ] Manufacturing
- [ ] Supply
- [ ] Storage
- [ ] Availability
  - [ ] *Location*
  - [ ] *In stock*
  - [ ] *Timely access*
- [ ] Readiness for use
  - [ ] *Cleanliness*
  - [ ] *Working order*
  - [ ] *Maintained*
- [ ] Accuracy
- [ ] Reliability
- [ ] Safety
- [ ] Equipment Compatibility
  - [ ] *Electrical*
- [ ] Safety coding
  - [ ] *Colour*
  - [ ] *Device interconnection*
- [ ] Model of equipment
- [ ] Equipment Failure

DRUGS

- [ ] Prescribing abbreviated
- [ ] Prescribing illegible
- [ ] Prescribing wrong drug
- [ ] Prescribing wrong dose
- [ ] Prescribing wrong frequency
- [ ] Interactions between drugs
- [ ] Duplication
- [ ] Multiple charts
- [ ] Ambiguity
  - [ ] *Dispensing*
  - [ ] *Preparation*
  - [ ] *Administer*
- [ ] Wrong patient
- [ ] Wrong drug
- [ ] Wrong route
- [ ] Time delay
- [ ] Frequency
  - [ ] *Too frequent*
  - [ ] *Too infrequent*
- [ ] Wrong dose
- [ ] Wrong equipment
- [ ] Wrong technique

CONSUMABLES
- [ ] Sterility
- [ ] Shelf life
- [ ] Administer
  - [ ] *Wrong patient*
  - [ ] *Wrong consumable*
  - [ ] *Incompatible*
  - [ ] *Left in patient*

NON CONSUMABLES
- [ ] Bed design
- [ ] Bed mechanical failure
- [ ] Bed electrical failure
- [ ] Bed mattress problem
- [ ] Bedrails
- [ ] Shower curtains
- [ ] Other

Figure 1.3 The SHEEP sheet.

Human Interaction

TEAM DYNAMICS & CONFLICT

PROBLEMS WITH TEAM
- [ ] Personality types
- [ ] Unclear team roles
- [ ] Preferred team role
- [ ] Perceived unfairness
- [ ] Perceived vs actual power
- [ ] Accountability
- [ ] Approach to change
- [ ] Difference in preferred communication styles
- [ ] Difference in preferred learning styles
- [ ] Mixed messages
- [ ] Preconceived ideas
- [ ] Conflicting expectations
- [ ] Skill mix

PROBLEMS WITH
- [ ] Patient interaction
- [ ] Conflict visibility
  - [ ] *Observable*
  - [ ] *Hidden*

PROBLEMS WITH LEADER
- [ ] Leadership styles
- [ ] Lack of leadership
- [ ] Lack of followership
- [ ] Hierarchy too steep
- [ ] Hierarchy too flat

BEHAVIOURS

INTERACTION QUALITY
- [ ] Challenging (negative) behaviour
- [ ] Lack of diversity consideration (gender, sex, culture, age)
- [ ] Prejudice
- [ ] Aggression
- [ ] Laziness
- [ ] Rudeness
- [ ] Snobbery
- [ ] Dishonesty
- [ ] Lack of consideration
- [ ] Lack of respect
  - [ ] *of others*
  - [ ] *by others*
- [ ] Over familiarity
- [ ] Empire building
- [ ] Trying to impress
- [ ] Negative responses
- [ ] Loss of sense of humour
- [ ] Unwillingness
- [ ] Apathy
- [ ] Fear
- [ ] Insecurity
- [ ] Making assumptions
- [ ] Reluctance to change
- [ ] Malicious intent

PROBLEMS WITH COMMUNICATION QUALITY
- [ ] Encoding
- [ ] Delivery
- [ ] Receipt
- [ ] Decoding
- [ ] Clarification
- [ ] Duplication
- [ ] Ambiguity
- [ ] Listening ability (receiving)
- [ ] Body language (non verbal)

PROBLEM WITH USER INTERACTION WITH EQUIPMENT
- [ ] Knowledge/Skill
  - [ ] *Training*
  - [ ] *Experience*
  - [ ] *Frequency of use*
  - [ ] *Familiarity*
  - [ ] *Ability to troubleshoot*
- [ ] Personal preference for equipment
- [ ] Availability of back-up equipment
- [ ] Ergonomic design/layout
  - [ ] *User Interface*
  - [ ] *Ease of Use*
  - [ ] *Complexity*
  - [ ] *Readability*
- [ ] Processing information
- [ ] Acting on information
- [ ] Post procedures check

INSTRUMENTS
- [ ] Sterility
- [ ] Administer
  - [ ] *Wrong patient*
  - [ ] *Wrong instrument*
  - [ ] *Incompatible*
  - [ ] *Left in patient*

MEDICAL GASES
- [ ] Prescribing
- [ ] Administer
  - [ ] *Wrong patient*
  - [ ] *Wrong gas*
  - [ ] *Wrong delivery method*
  - [ ] *Wrong time*
  - [ ] *Wrong dose*

HUMAN TISSUE, BLOOD PRODUCTS & TRANSPLANTATION
- [ ] Collection
- [ ] Processing
- [ ] Prescribing
- [ ] Preparation
  - [ ] *Cross matching*
  - [ ] *Other preparation*
- [ ] Administer
  - [ ] *Wrong patient*
  - [ ] *Wrong blood/ Product/organ*
  - [ ] *Wrong route*
  - [ ] *Wrong time*
    - [ ] *Point*
    - [ ] *Delay*
    - [ ] *Duration*
- [ ] Wrong dose

- [ ] Patient monitor failure

IMPLANTS / PROSTHESES
- [ ] Functionality
- [ ] Insertion

Environment

LOCATION CHANGE

PROBLEMS WITH JOURNEY BETWEEN LOCATIONS
- [ ] Complexity
- [ ] Distance
- [ ] Accessibility
  - [ ] *Size*
  - [ ] *Secure areas*
- [ ] Modality of transfer
  - [ ] *Foot*
  - [ ] *Chair*
  - [ ] *Trolley/bed/stretcher*
  - [ ] *Vehicle*
  - [ ] *Lift/elevator*
  - [ ] *Lifting device (Hoist)*

INTERRUPTIONS
- [ ] People
- [ ] Equipment, Bleep
- [ ] Phones
- [ ] Machines
- [ ] Media (text, email)

PHYSICAL PROBLEMS WITH
- [ ] Atmospheric composition (air)
- [ ] Temperature
- [ ] Humidity
- [ ] Smell
- [ ] Lighting
- [ ] Noise
- [ ] Cleanliness
- [ ] Size
- [ ] Security
- [ ] Tidiness

ERGONOMICS

PHYSICAL DESIGN PROBLEMS WITH
- [ ] Infrastructure (walls etc)
- [ ] Immovable structures (cupboards)
- [ ] Movable structures (beds, chairs)

TASK RELATED DESIGN PROBLEMS WITH
- [ ] Resource location
- [ ] Knowing where it is
- [ ] Visibility
- [ ] Accessible
- [ ] Organised
- [ ] Standardised
- [ ] Optimised

SAFETY CONTROLS
- [ ] Radiation
- [ ] Electromagnetic field (eg MRI, laser)
- [ ] Biochemical hazard

FUNCTIONAL DESIGN PROBLEMS WITH
- [ ] Proximity to eating/ resting/physiological function areas
- [ ] Privacy

VICINITY
- [ ] Arms reach area
- [ ] Immediate vicinity (no doors)
- [ ] Departmental area
- [ ] Hospital/GP practice/ Clinical unit
- [ ] External

of your SHEEP on a daily basis, it is possible to become aware of when we are more likely to make a mistake and institute the extra checking behaviours we will cover later. The factors involved will be constantly changing. We need to promote risk awareness in order to make our patients safer. It involves a change of mind set. As with any new skill, it is necessary to practise. Please try Example 1.1 using the SHEEP sheet.

Example 1.1 Please use the SHEEP sheet for the following real-life examples

It was after midnight. It was an emergency case. Only junior staff were in the hospital, the senior staff were now in bed and on call from home. A new junior anaesthetist who was keen and competent had seen the patient and had performed a preoperative visit. The surgeon and the anaesthetist had not worked together before. Both doctors had already been working for over 16 hours.

The patient was an intravenous drug user who required an incision and drainage of groin abscess. It took over 30 minutes to establish intravenous access (a small piece of plastic inserted with a needle that goes into a vein enabling drugs to be given). The process of regularly using veins to insert illicit drugs damages the veins over time. Finally, with a sense of triumph and relief, a small vein midway along the inner aspect of the forearm was located. It was only a 24G cannula (a very small blue drip). The induction of anaesthesia (putting the patient to sleep) was uneventful. The patient was transferred to theatre.

When the surgeon made the incision into the 'abscess' it became apparent that all was not as it seemed. The diagnosis was not in fact an abscess at all but instead a femoral artery aneurysm (a ballooning of a blood vessel that can occur following drug use). The blood was pulsing out at high pressure. The artery was crumbling in front of the surgeon's eyes. What should have been a simple procedure was fast becoming a major haemorrhage (large amount of blood lost).

The surgeon could not stop the bleeding. The anaesthetist only had a small drip through which they could not replace the fluid lost fast enough. The patient quickly became haemodynamically unstable (blood pressure dropped below safe levels).

Both the anaesthetist and the surgeon called for senior help.

The scrub team and the surgeon attempted to pack the wound and just put pressure on it. The situation resembled the Dutch boy with his finger in the dyke. The vascular surgeon was travelling in from home.

The registrar in anaesthesia had been closer to hand and had run from Intensive Care. Following a struggle and multiple attempts, they managed to secure central access through a track in the neck (a different type of drip into a big vein in the neck where the patient had used their own veins). This allowed faster administration of fluids and drugs.

The consultant vascular surgeon had to perform a laparotomy (a big cut across the abdomen, major surgery) whilst the only access at this time was still the small blue cannula.

A clamp was placed on a large artery in the abdomen. From this time onwards it was possible to recover the situation.

The patient spent the next day on the Intensive Care and made a full recovery albeit with a large, unexpected abdominal wound.

How many contributory factors can you identify?

A few things to consider:

◆ Time of day. Errors are more likely at night.

◆ Length of shift. Errors are more likely with fatigue.

◆ System error. Shift lengths should be limited by the European Working Time Directive.

◆ Junior staff. Less experienced. Often unsupervised at night or supervised from home.

◆ Unfamiliar team.

◆ Unfamiliar hospital. Unfamiliar theatre. Unfamiliar with protocols and systems.

◆ Diagnosis confirmed only by one team member. Not checked or questioned by another.

◆ Assumption. A regular occurrence in errors. The anaesthetist did not question the surgical diagnosis. They made an assumption that it was an abscess.

◆ There is an assumption that a surgically simple case will be paralleled by a 'simple' anaesthetic.

◆ 'Just a quick anaesthetic' is a phrase that has preceded many a disaster.

◆ Patient factors making the case more difficult in a number of ways.

◆ Systems and protocols are in place to reduce out-of-hours operating.

More learning points:

Things are not always what they seem.

Always ask yourself:

'What else could this be?'

'What are we missing here?'

'Am I making an assumption?'

Now try Example 1.2.

Example 1.2 Please use the SHEEP sheet

Mrs D was a fit and healthy 46-year-old who attended her GP with frequency (passing urine more often than usual). Following a urine dipstick she was treated with antibiotics. The results of the urine sample (M, C, and S—microscopy, culture, and sensitivity, i.e. taking a urine sample and looking at it under a microscope and trying to see whether there are bacteria present and if so, which antibiotics would kill them) were not followed up.

Mrs D was really no better but had a very uncomplaining personality and so struggled on. The symptoms persisted and she returned a few weeks later to the GP. On this occasion she saw a different doctor but the story was the same. A urine sample and some more antibiotics. No resolution but in fact a worsening of symptoms.

Mrs D really didn't like to make a fuss. She never normally saw her doctor but returned to the GP a third time and a fourth time and a fifth time over the course of 4 months. She had started to notice some blood in her urine.

She decided, following the insistence of her more assertive sister, to attend the Emergency department following a larger amount of haematuria (blood in the urine). With a urine sample taken, she was sent home with yet another dose of antibiotics. 'It's just a UTI [urinary tract infection]. Take these and you'll be right as rain in a few days!'

A further GP visit and another trip to the Emergency department and two more doses of antibiotics later, there was a new symptom. Having been falsely reassured for over 7 months, Mrs D presented with a lymph node swelling in her right thigh. A diagnosis of advanced bladder cancer was made.

Despite chemotherapy, bilateral nephrostomy tubes (tubes that go into both of your kidneys through your back so the urine goes out of the body in a different way than through your bladder), radiotherapy, and surgery, it was all too late. The tumour was too advanced.

The irony of the statement, 'If only we could have started the treatment sooner' should not be missed.

Mrs D died with a bladder cancer and a fungating lymph node (cancer in the lymph node grew out through her skin). She left behind three children, the youngest of whom was only 10 years old.

Mrs D was my friend. We let her down.

One of the things that was emphasized repeatedly when I was a medical student was 'common things are common'. Of course, this is true for a population but may not help the individual. At what stage do we question ourselves? What else could this be? What am I missing here? Do I agree with the current working diagnosis? This common thing is not behaving in a common way, what else could it be? Am I asking the right questions?

What about the quality of the information transfer? How often do you ask yourself, 'Have I got all of the information?'.

Did any of the doctors have the big picture or was each event treated in isolation? How was the information transfer within the general practice? Was there adequate information exchange between secondary and primary care?

Did the gentle nature of the patient who was neither demanding nor assertive affect the outcome? How should we alter our management to ensure we are approachable and empower our patients to feel able to challenge us?

How hard was it to look my friend's family in the eye when we stood in the kitchen as she lay resting upstairs in the final days of her life and they asked me, 'Why?'.

Please try Example 1.3.

Example 1.3 Non-clinical example—post interview

There was an interview for a senior nursing position. The candidates were not informed immediately after the interviews who had been successful. They were told they would hear the following day.

The next morning, the appointed candidate was informed of their success and proceeded to send an email to their senior colleagues within the organization to inform them. One of these colleagues was a close friend to a rival candidate. They quickly text their friend to offer support in a 'better luck next time' format. The candidate had not yet been told about the outcome of the interview.

It is not only harm to patients that I am keen to avoid. Our staff are central to everything we do and we need to get better at caring for them too. There is clear evidence that staff moral has a direct impact on the quality of patient care. We must get better at looking after ourselves in order to get better at looking after our patients.

Example 1.4 is another one to try.

Example 1.4 Information flow and system errors

A senior registrar in haematology was planning to teach a junior colleague how to perform a bone marrow biopsy under local anaesthetic and sedation. The two doctors discussed the theory of the procedure in the treatment room while drawing up both the local anaesthetic (10mL of 1% lignocaine) and the sedative (10mL of midazolam) in two separate syringes. Both drugs in syringes were then placed in a tray along with all the other equipment required to perform the biopsy. The doctors left the treatment room and went to the patient.

The first step of the procedure was to insert intravenous access (a drip). Having prepared the trolley with all the equipment, obtained informed consent, and attached some simple monitoring, it was time to start. It is usual practice to have two doctors: one for the procedure and one for the sedation.

The next step was to give the sedative drug.

'Give 2 mL', said the senior registrar.

'OK, 2mL in,' replied the SHO (senior house officer).

'How are you feeling there Mr Brown? Noticed any difference?'

Mr Brown said he felt completely normal and had not noticed any changes at all.

'Give another 2mL.'

'OK, another 2mL in.'

'Which syringe are you using? Oh my God! You idiot! That's the wrong drug! Give me the other syringe!'

4mg of midazolam now administered.

Procedure was completed uneventfully from that point onwards.

The intravenous lignocaine caused no ill effects.

So let's try to identify our layers of cheese. It is great that there was an attempt at a briefing before the procedure started. This should be routine and should involve a conversation about potential risks, starting to look for the errors in advance. What should not happen is that you should not be talking while you are drawing up drugs. I have observed a marked difference in how the medical and nursing professions are taught when it comes to drug preparation. I am not proud to admit that I have witnessed anything from no training whatsoever to a rather blasé attitude bordering on cavalier within the medical fraternity. My personal experience is shared in Example 1.5.

There are emerging pockets of excellence with regard to drug preparation and we will return to this in a future chapter. Trying to multitask (talking and preparing the drug at the same time) as in Example 1.4 would not fulfil these higher standards of care.

The syringes in Example 1.4 were not labelled and no attempt was made to distinguish between the two. No difference in size of the syringe. No difference in volume in the syringes. No difference in the colour of the needle attached. No attempt to isolate the two drugs in different containers and keep them with the ampoules from which they were drawn up. No visual cues at all as to which drug was where. This was an error waiting to happen with no risk awareness.

There was no clear communication between the doctors at the bedside as to which drug was to be given. The drugs were not named as part of the instruction.

Using pronouns, such as give 'it', has been the source of a number of major errors. Communication should follow a set pattern including confirmation of the drug name, drug dose in mg, and volume of drug to be given. No further checking of ampoules took place as they had been disposed of in the treatment room.

On this occasion it was fortunate that a small dose of intravenous lignocaine (a local anaesthetic which has a relatively good safety profile) did not cause harm. Had it been a different local anaesthetic injected into the vein, the story could have been very different.

The response to the discovery of the error was also less than ideal. There is no excuse for poor behaviour even within a crisis and in front of a patient is even less excusable. The patient was entitled to an explanation, not simply a large dose of sedation with an amnesic effect. We need to move towards a system of error management that becomes routine.

Example 1.5 is a personal example of how underprepared I felt when first on the wards. I had not been trained for the tasks I was expected to perform.

Osmosis seemed to be a common teacher whilst I was a medical student and a trainee. It is, however, rather too random a trainer for my liking. I would like to put my hand on my heart and say that the training is so much better now. When I run simulation sessions for medical students and foundation trainees,

---

Example 1.5 Personal example

On my first week on the wards (admittedly 20 years ago), I was informed that none of the nurses on that shift had their 'IV certificate' as someone had gone off sick. (This is like a driving licence for drawing up and delivering drugs into a cannula/drip that nurses took but doctors did not.) This meant it was down to me to give all of the 'IV's. The problem was that I had no training whatsoever in drawing up or giving of these drugs. On requesting help from my team, I was basically told to 'feel free to cope!'. I admit that I used a degree of common sense and gathered all the information I could from the resources available. The Oxford handbook which lived in my white coat pocket was not terribly helpful on this subject (this was well before the times of bare below the elbows and our friend Google). I read the packets in the drug boxes and hoped for the best.

Fortunately, on this occasion, other than spraying myself with an antibiotic as I mistimed the extraction of the air through the rubber bung, no harm ensued.

---

there are still a significant number who can neither mix up an intravenous drug nor run though a giving set (set up a drip) as no one has ever taken the time to show them. Neither task is difficult or complicated but the latter task may be necessary in a hurry one day in a case of anaphylaxis or haemorrhage. In that emergency setting is surely not the best time to be doing a task for the first time.

The examples so far begin to hint at the complexity of how the layers of cheese can start to line up. In the next five chapters we will consider each of the letters of SHEEP in turn in order to focus on what goes wrong in a more structured way.

Key points

◆ To err is human.

◆ We need to embed an open culture.

◆ There should be an inquisitive approach to error that seeks out the learning and shares it.

◆ The new error checklist—the SHEEP sheet—helps gather more information following an event or a near miss. It is quick and easy to use.

◆ Things are not always what they seem: avoid assumption.

◆ 'What am I missing here?' is a healthy question to keep asking.

◆ We need to give the right training to the right people at the right time in their career path.

References

1. Reason J. Understanding adverse events: human factors. *Quality & Safety in Health Care* 1995;4(2):80–9.
2. Reason J. Human error: models and management. *British Medical Journal* 2000;320(7237):768–70.
3. Reason J. Beyond the organisational accident: the need for 'error wisdom' on the front-line. *Quality & Safety in Health Care* 2004;13(Suppl 2):ii28–33.
4. Jeffs L, Berta W, Lingard L, Baker GR. Learning from near misses: from quick fixes to closing off the Swiss-cheese holes. *BMJ Quality & Safety* 2012;21(4):287–94.
5. Molloy GJ, O'Boyle CA. The SHEL model: a useful tool for analyzing and teaching the contribution of human factors to medical error. *Academic Medicine* 2005;80(2):152–5.
6. Martin P, Turner B. Grounded theory and organizational research. *The Journal of Behavioral Science* 1986;22(2):141–57.

7. Li W, Liu K, Li S, Yang H. Normative modeling for personalized clinical pathway using organizational semiotics methods. *International Symposium on Computer Science and Computational Technology* 2008:3–7.

8. Gawande A. The checklist: if something so simple can transform intensive care, what else can it do? *New Yorker* 2007:86–101.

9. Gawande A. Checklists for success inside the OR and beyond: an interview with Atul Gawanda, MD, FACS. Interview by Tony Peregrin. *Bulletin of the American College of Surgeons* 2010;95(5):24–7.

10. Haynes AB, Weiser TG, Berry WR, Lipsitz SR, Breizat AH, Dellinger EP, *et al.* A surgical safety checklist to reduce morbidity and mortality in a global population. *New England Journal of Medicine* 2009;360(5):491–9.

2

The 'S' of SHEEP: Systems

Experience is the name every one gives to their mistakes

Oscar Wilde, 1854–1900
Lady Windermere's Fan (1892), Act 3

Introduction

Let's start by exploring the 'S' of the algorithm (see Figure 2.1).

Formal versus Informal

Within healthcare there is a huge number of formal published procedures and then far more informal unwritten processes that are culturally ingrained or learnt in an 'osmosis'-style apprenticeship. It is this invisible 'culture', which is interleaved with science, knowledge, and skills, that strongly influences our behaviours. When I began to explore some of the processes that exist within hospitals I was met with a wide variety of responses. The replies included, 'That is just how we do it here!' or 'I don't really know why we do it like that, we just do!' or 'I've always done it that way'. Culture will form the substance of a future chapter. For now we will focus on the more formal systems, beginning with information.

Information

It is necessary to consider information and its flow as a key part of any organization. This flow of information is often termed 'communication' but I wish to reserve that term for something different.

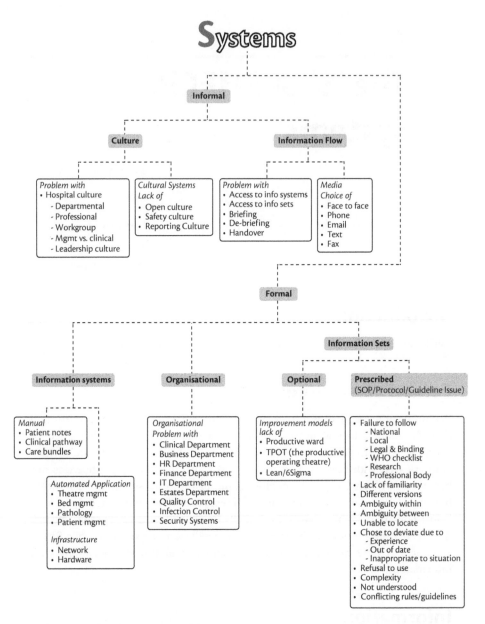

Figure 2.1 'S'—the SHEEP model.

I would like you to consider the information itself (**information sets**), where the information is stored (**information systems**), and also how the information moves about or is transferred (**information flow**). We should also consider the user of the information and how they can interact with each of the information sets, systems, and flow.

Information sets

Policies, policies, and more policies

Within the NHS we work with enormous numbers of processes, protocols, policies, standard operating procedures (SOPs), care pathways, care bundles, and guidelines.

Formal SOPs

For ease, in the book I will use SOP to refer to all of the formal terms just listed (i.e. written documents that describe a series of actions. The actions can be suggestions or compulsory).

The formal SOPs can be published at a national level, a regional level, or a local level. They are published by government agencies, professional bodies, specialist interest groups, journals, hospitals, or departments. There can be ambiguity between the different sources of the SOP or even between different versions of the same policy (some real-life examples are included in Examples 2.1–2.4).

> ## Example 2.1 SOP example
>
> There were six versions of a Falls policy found on one ward at the same time. Not surprisingly, the nursing staff were using different ones on different patients and sometimes even on the same patient. It would be fair to say that there was confusion and a higher chance of an error occurring. The earlier versions of the policy were considered to be missing vital steps that would keep our patients safe. The patients that were, therefore, being cared for using the incorrect earlier version were missing out from this vital learning.

> ## Example 2.2 Further SOP example
>
> A labour ward was using a local policy to define the urgency of the caesarean sections which was different from the national definitions. Confusion arose regularly between the two systems among anaesthetists, obstetricians, and midwifery staff. The consequence was miscommunication about the urgency of some caesarean sections resulting in a decreased standard of care and delays in getting a patient to theatre.

Example 2.3 Ambiguity

There comes a time in anaesthesia when you are a trainee, having worked on the Intensive Care Unit, that you are deemed 'experienced' with inotropes (a type of drug used to help the heart to pump blood around the body). This point of adequate experience is not clearly defined. During the time before you reach this informal level you should use the anaphylaxis (potentially life-threatening allergic reaction) guidelines from the Resuscitation Council UK. After this informal moment (currently left to the individual to decide), you can use a different guideline from the Association of Anaesthetists. The question is, when are you deemed experienced with inotropes? There is no assessment. Are you to use the Resuscitation Council guidelines one day and the next you have graduated to using the Association guidelines? I have been asked this question on several occasions during simulation training. It is a tricky one to answer. I'm not sure that in the middle of an episode of anaphylaxis is the best time for ambiguity.

Example 2.4 More Ambiguity

A new drug chart has been introduced in a hospital that has a code of both letters and numbers. The letters are used to explain possible different routes of administration. The numbers are used to explain the different options as to why it may be necessary to deviate from the prescription (e.g. nil by mouth, when the patient is waiting for elective surgery).

However, there is an 'S' to represent that the patient took their drugs them'S'elf and a number '5' which is then used to refer to a more detailed part of the chart where an explanation for not giving the drug is written out in full. When an S and a 5 are handwritten they can look extremely similar and cause confusion.

On one occasion the anaesthetist was pleased that the patient had taken their beta-blocker themSelf on the morning of surgery. An S was thought to be entered on the drug chart. This group of drugs can be used for the treatment of high blood pressure and tends to stop the heart beating too quickly. The drugs seem to confer an advantage when taken before an anaesthetic. However, it was a 5 and the nurse on that particular ward round was unaware that giving the drug even when the patient is 'nil by mouth' is best for the patient. It is a common source of confusion as ideas on the topic are constantly changing. The patient had an episode of a very fast heart rate following the start of the anaesthetic. Fortunately on this occasion no harm came to the patient but it is important that we learn from everything and try and make the system safer.

So is the error the fault of the person writing the SOP or the person using the SOP? The idea of 'fault' is something that we are trying to move away from. The answer is one of shared responsibility. The writer has a responsibility to make the SOP as clear as possible. If the user is unsure then they have a responsibility to seek clarification.

Let's try to improve our writing of SOPs (see Box 2.1).

Box 2.1 So what makes an effective SOP?

◆ People need to know it exists.

◆ There should only be one version available.

◆ Staff need to be able to locate it easily.

◆ It needs to be short, ideally one side of A4.

◆ It should be clear to the most junior of the users.

◆ The style, font, colour scheme, and design of the document should be carefully planned.

◆ The author's name should be printed on the document.

◆ The version should be clearly documented.

◆ The date for next review of the document should be clear.

◆ A source for more detail or background information should be included.

Let's look at each of those points in turn.

People need to know the SOP exists

As an aside, I would like you to consider, 'How do you know what you do not know?'.

There is a theory surrounding this, which if you would like to consider further you can look up 'Johari window'.

We all have a blind spot of the 'unknown unknown'.

A member of staff will not follow a SOP if they do not know it exists. One of the problems is that SOPs can be produced by such a large variety of sources and then distributed via a wide choice of differing media. Due to the differing way that we personally prefer to receive information, we make choices about how others might wish to receive it. Have you considered your own preferences? If you are to receive new information would you like: email, a PowerPoint presentation, face to face, written information, if so, would you prefer colourful or black and white, with or without charts and data, perhaps you would prefer to attend a conference or a course, read a journal, see a poster campaign, website . . . ? There is no single approach that will suit all styles. If you are the one attempting to deliver information, for example, to alert people to the existence of a new guideline, remember to employ a mixture of approaches. Caution: see Box 2.2.

Box 2.2 Warning—soapbox moment

The topic of how ineffectual I consider email to be will occur more than once. The most important thing to remember is that sending an email does not mean that your message has been received, let alone understood.

I digress, back to SOPs.

There should only be one version of the SOP available

Both ambiguity and variation can be sources of error.

If there are six versions of the same falls policy on a ward, how should the staff know which one they are supposed to be using? If there is a difference between the SOP from a professional body and one produced locally, which should they use and how will they know about the two versions?

I have yet to fully understand when a guideline exists at a national level why we find the need to rewrite a local version. I can understand the thought that by making a process feel like it is locally driven or owned it may be possible to influence people more quickly to adopt the change. However, I can see far more downsides to this approach. The NHS workforce is not static. Trainee medical staff rotate through hospitals annually or often even more frequently. We use a large pool of agency or locum staff who may work at different hospitals. Huge amounts of research, expert panels, and Cochrane reviews are undertaken to try and establish 'best practice'. Why would you want to deviate from the best?

When I talk about standardization, I am sometimes accused of removing professionalism in decision-making or replacing years of training with a menial checklist.

My answer: over the tannoy you hear the following, 'Ladies and gentleman, your captain today has decided that he has been flying for over 20 years and so he has decided to do all your pre-flight checks from memory. He is confident that as he has been doing it so long, he can probably remember all of them most of the time . . . '. Would you stay on the plane?

Human beings are fallible. There is nothing more certain than that all of us will make mistakes. Why is it not culturally accepted that there is no harm in double checking? There is safety in admitting our vulnerability. We will return to double checking later as even how we do the double checking is important.

Staff need to be able to locate the SOP easily

I would like to introduce the concept of mental workload, a concept we will revisit later in more detail. For now, I would like you to consider examples of when this may occur including: performing a complex task or a task where there is a high degree of emotional overlay, or an emergency setting when there is a time pressure or a lack of familiarity with task/environment, or a situation when trying to plan and prioritize multiple tasks.

When you are already functioning under a high workload, it may be advantageous to locate a SOP as quickly as possible. If the system used to access the SOP is slow or complex, it acts as a disincentive to follow the right behaviour (i.e. to locate the SOP and use it).

The SOP may be in paper format or located in some form of electronic media. We use the term information system to refer to this format.

The SOP needs to be short, ideally one side of A4

Blaise Pascal (French mathematician, physicist, 1623–1662) wrote in 1657,[1] 'I have made this letter longer than normal, because I lack the time to make it shorter' (*Lettres provinciales*, letter XVI).

I would describe the current culture in parts of the NHS as 'time poor' and 'fire fighting'. In fact, on the results of our early work with the SHEEP sheet the categories that were ticked most frequently by NHS staff as contributing to error were 'time pressure' and 'high workload'.

This enormous time pressure is due to a number of factors including lack of resources, inadequate staffing levels, and inappropriate skill mix. The net result is a lack of time to think. How often in your working day can you just stop and t–h–i–n–k?

I believe that it is this lack of time that means we do not have the time to really focus on what we are saying in the SOP. It tends to end up overcomplicated. It takes time and a deeper understanding to only list a summary of the most salient points (a clear signpost to a fuller version can always be included in the document).

It is also the fact that we are time poor that feeds our need for SOPs to be focused and to the point. We don't have the time to wade through lengthy and complicated SOPs. When you are under pressure, this simply becomes frustrating as you skim read trying to find the bit you need. This increases the chance of error.

The SOP should be clear to the most junior of the users

The language used should be free from jargon and should not contain abbreviations. All technical terms should be explained and no assumptions made about baseline knowledge levels.

The language should be clean and not open to misinterpretation or ambiguity.

A good safety check is a review by the target audience. In addition, apply the 6-year-old child or alien test (i.e. if I was explaining this to either of these, would they understand?) Aim for a 'Noddy's guide'. (For those of you who are too young, or didn't grow up in the UK, Noddy was a character in a children's series of books and later on television while I was growing up. It has colloquially come to mean a very simplified version, suitable for child-like understanding.)

I am a firm believer in the old cliché that a picture speaks a thousand words, so consider including a pictorial representation of the process if you can.

How the SOP is actually displayed is also relevant. The colour, the layout, and the font style and size will affect how well the information is taken in, processed, and understood. Remember also that people approach written information differently. For example, if you present people with several lists of information displayed in columns, some people will read down the lists whilst others will read across. There are guidelines published by Gawande[2,3] on how to write a checklist. There is a whole area of research looking at design of posters, information, and marketing on how to best grab our attention and maximize the impact the material has (this is beyond the scope of this book).

Pilot your SOP with a large sample of the people who will be using it. Empower them to alter it by giving them a red pen or encourage them to track changes (this parallels teachers and homework). Think about the language you use to really encourage them to give you honest feedback.

The author's name should be printed on the document

Inclusion of the author's name allows a point of contact in case clarification is required and also someone to keep track of versions and updates as appropriate.

The version should be clearly documented

It is helpful to know which version you have in your hand. In Example 2.1, I would need to locate Falls Version 6.0. The previous versions should be removed as the new one arrives!

The author needs to continue to monitor changes in the field, not just write the SOP and wash their hands of it. There needs to be a commitment to stay up to date with a strong evidence base if available and failing that, at least a good dose of common sense.

The date for next review of the document should be clear

Along the bottom of one side of A4, next to the author and the version number, should be a review date for the SOP to be updated and compared to best practice.

A source for more detailed/background information should be included

This fulfils more than one purpose. Firstly, a longer version can include information concerning more unusual circumstances or more complex situations. It can also serve to fulfil the needs for those with certain learning styles to read the theory behind something before accepting it.

And so my plea is that you write the long, archaic version of the policy if you must. But please, also write a short, punchy one-side summary of the key points following the simple rules given earlier.

Information systems

Within information sets, we have started to consider different ways of storing information including paper and electronic media. Let's start with paper.

Whilst paper may sound a little old fashioned, there are some advantages. Paper is portable which may be useful if you want to take the information to the patient's bedside in an emergency. Paper is cheap (relative to buying a PC, tablet, or mobile technology) but does have 'green' costs. If a new version of the SOP is created someone needs to remove all of the old versions and replace them with the new version. This system is reliant on a human remembering to perform this step and perhaps it may affect a number of clinical areas. If you are responsible for a change in a version of a policy, remember the possible flaws in this step. Where and how the paper version is stored needs consideration. We have mentioned accessibility. Within this concept we need to consider the storage system. Is the paper stored in files/shelves/drawers? Is there a logical and systematic way to find everything—using alphabetical order or colour coding? Is the technique standardized, e.g. are all the wards using the same method?

Access to electronic media requires a systems-based approach too. Are there adequate numbers of user interfaces (PCs, tablets, smart phones, mobile computers)? When the device is turned on, how long does it take to warm up? What would happen in a life-threatening, time-critical emergency when the computer takes minutes to warm up and yet every wasted second could make a difference? Once the computer is on how many button presses does it take to find the emergency protocols? Are they all grouped together in a clearly marked site that could not be missed or misinterpreted? Is there training for all new staff and are there regular updates for current staff? Has the system been checked for usability with the lowest common denominator of users who have the least IT skills? Is there a reliable, available source of help to troubleshoot? Is there a maintenance programme and adequate financial provision for updating systems in the future? Do all of the various electronic systems talk to each other? Is there one login for all of the data? Is it secure? Secure firstly from a data protection standpoint. Would it stand up to the scrutiny of the governance systems and the Caldicott guardian? But also secure that no patient or, sadly, staff would like to take the electronic gizmo home with them, and yes, it has happened.

Information flow

Publicizing information across an organization as large as a hospital is challenging, let alone trying to share information across the whole NHS. The NHS is exceedingly guilty of 'left hand not knowing the actions of right hand syndrome'. Even within one hospital gaps of information flow can occur between management and clinical staff, between nurses and doctors and vice versa, between seniors and juniors, between professions, and between disciplines. Improving this information flow is critical to success within a hospital and by 'success', I mean safe and high-quality care.

I call the following model for information flow '*Debbie's Diamond*'. It is diamond in shape but should also represent the fact that good information flow requires clarity and is hard! (I hope also that you will wonder if at times my tongue may be in my cheek.)

As part of encouraging culture change we need to tackle the steep hierarchy that exists across the NHS and flatten it off a bit. I mention this here as I wish to move away from the concepts of 'top-down' and 'bottom-up' approaches to management structure and instead view information flow as going 'across' an organization.

The traditional approach is to draw a triangle with the management at the top. This positioning at the top helps to keep that hierarchy alive and well. I have used the abbreviation CEO for the chief executive officer.

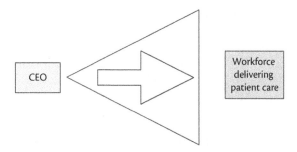

Figure 2.2 Traditional organizational diagram rotated through 90 degrees.

By rotating the triangle, it is possible to view things differently (see Figure 2.2).

Adopting the default in the Western world to read a page from left to right, it is now possible to think of information flowing across an organization from left to right.

However, information flow must be two-way. By placing a mirror to the right of the triangle we can see a diamond. The right-hand side represents the flow of information back from the workforce delivering patient care towards the CEO (see Figure 2.3).

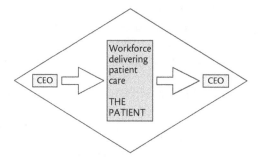

Figure 2.3 Information flow across management structure and feedback to close the communication loop.

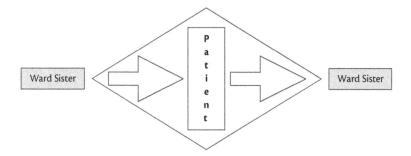

Figure 2.4 Diamond model at local ward level.

In the Diamond model the majority of the workforce is within the centre of the diamond as they represent both the largest numbers but are also central to the success of the organization. This layer is often referred to as 'shop floor', 'coal face', or 'sharp end'. My approach prefers to think of the patient being central to everything that we do. The care should be 'patient centric' and those closest to the patient who should also be 'central' to everything we do.

The diamond can represent any level of information flow, for example, starting with a ward sister and spreading across the ward to include all bands of nursing staff, allied health professionals such as physiotherapists, occupational therapists, dieticians, pharmacists, and non-clinical staff such as ward clerks, porters, and cleaners, and, of course, to the **patients themselves**. All the staff groups are sharing their roles and expertise and explanations with the patient. This helps to be honest about what we can achieve and helps to blend realism with patient expectations.

There is a stage of **listening** and **asking** questions.

How often do we really listen to our patients and give them the time they need? We need to establish what the patient needs/would like/expects. It would be useful to gather their ideas and suggestions and feedback.

Our patients should not be aware of the time pressure we are under. If, however, you will not return to them for 10 minutes or 20 minutes, then be honest. Don't use the throwaway phrases, 'I'll be right back' or 'I'll be back in a minute'. I am a strong believer in a smile and an upbeat affect too. If we have systems that interfere with the time that we can give to our patients, it is time to change the systems. Once we have established our patients' needs, we can pass that information on.

Information flow then returns from the bedside through any of those groups already mentioned to the ward sister or charge nurse (see Figure 2.4). But at each stage we can alter our delivery of care to tailor make it to our patients. By this process we have a continuous feedback on quality of care and a chance to adjust it as we go along (see Figure 2.5).

Information flow needs to become continuous (see Figure 2.5).

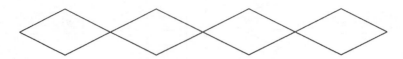

Figure 2.5 The diagram shows how the end of one diamond becomes the start of the next.

The process should be one of continuous 'tweaking' following feedback so it is a 'continually responsive improvement' model that is patient centric and where the patient is truly involved in influencing their care.

The last important thing is the interaction to transfer the information **must** *be face to face (**not** email!).*

So what sort of information can flow in this way?

I would propose a framework based on the rule of three (human brains generally work well with a three grouping). It should be focused and specific. An example (Table 2.1) is included for a ward-level discussion.

So looking at Table 2.1, can you work out the sample information framework? (For the generic framework see Table 2.2)

There is a pattern of **big picture, praise, and local** grouped in three.

The praise should not be last as it should not be a throwaway comment at the end. It is also the opposite of the sandwich style of feedback that many are familiar with across the NHS. So often the feedback is delivered in a 'positive–negative–positive' format. It has resulted in a Pavlovian response such that when some staff are praised, they ignore it and wait only for the criticism that

Table 2.1 Ward Level Discussion

This week's Trust focus is on DVT prophylaxis.
The Trust is currently running at 88% for our DVT rates which is just below our target of 90%.
What can we do in this ward to help that improve?
Praise (Trust wide)
Huge thanks go to the paediatric department for all of their hard work to make the CQC visit such a success.
Praise (local)
We would like to thank Doreen last week for working that extra shift at such short notice.
Local focus
We need a big push on using the new discharge lounge facility.
We missed our planned discharge times on four patients last week, resulting in failed admissions.
How can we make it better? Any ideas?

Table 2.2 Outward limb of information flow (left-hand side of diamond)

Trust focus
1. Aim
2. Data
3. Any suggestions?
Praise
◆ Trust
◆ Local
Local focus
1. Aim
2. Data
3. Any suggestions?

inevitably used to follow. The bread on either side of the sandwich is used to disguise the unpalatable taste of the filling. We will return to a whole chapter on giving feedback and debriefing in book 2.

Cliché alert: praise should be central to all that we do! There is evidence from Professor Michael West's group that receiving genuine specific praise can raise moral which in turn will increase performance.

The information that then returns from the department level back across the organization is fed into the next information flow cycle (see Box 2.3).

Box 2.3 Return information flow (right-hand side of diamond)

◆ Suggestions for improvement on Trust topic.

◆ Person to be nominated for Trust-wide/local praise.

◆ Suggestions for improvement on local topic (including patient suggestions!).

Each face-to-face meeting is a brief and debrief 'meeting'. Briefing and debriefing are important topics that deserve an in-depth review in book 2. Running effective meetings will also be covered there.

Let's return to systems and to Figure 2.1.

Informal—brief look at culture

There has been a large emphasis recently on moving towards a 'no blame' culture. I disagree. Harold Shipman should be blamed for his actions. Injecting insulin purposefully into a bag of fluid is an intentional act. There should be blame. I hope we can all agree these cases are clear cut.

For me, 'no blame' is a step too far. As I have mentioned, some institutions (including the Institute for Improvement) have adopted the term 'just culture'. I don't like that term either. For me, when we understand the role of clean language, the words 'just' and 'justice' are too close. A just culture for me goes too far back to the old ways implying an element of punishment and judgement.

I like the term 'open' culture. There are different strands which I feel are encompassed by this term. It implies that we will admit when we have made a mistake. We would be open to reporting it. We would embrace the learning that could follow. I am also happy with the term learning culture.

Yes, for those of you who are awake, some of the content of the last three paragraphs was discussed in the previous chapter. I have included some of it again for two reasons, firstly knowing that repetition is often required to ensure learning and secondly I'm also aware that some readers will start at Chapter 2. For those of you for whom it was not required, I hope you will forgive me!

What about wanton deviation from a protocol or SOP? This is something that is sometimes referred to as 'work arounds'. Is that OK?

What if they were arrogant and felt they were too important to follow the WHO checklist and then they were involved in a wrong-site surgery? Is that OK?

What if they made a clinical judgement that the protocol was not suitable for the patient's condition? Is that OK?

What if the protocol was considered to be out of date and this expert was aware of the new research? Is that OK?

What if they had been drinking that night and then they were called in from home? Is that OK? Would it matter if it was a mouthful? Or a glass? Or two or three? Who decides? Who would challenge them? And how? What if they were the only one with that expertise?

What if they had been drinking the night before and were not drunk now but clearly hung-over? Is that OK?

How are you making your decisions? Are these ethical and moral or cultural norms that we are exploring?

Some of these issues go beyond the informal boundaries of culture and acceptable norms. Some of these examples belong on the formal part of the algorithm, but how do you know which ones? Are you going to trust your gut instinct or their track record?

I think the most useful tool to help you formulate ideas in this type of setting is the incident decision tree (formerly available from the National Patient Safety Agency (NPSA) but this agency no longer exists). Have a go at using it on the examples in the previous couple of paragraphs (see Chapter 1, Figure 1.1).

There are definitely times when formal systems are appropriate. Let us start with one of these.

Legal

Negligence is for a judge to decide. I am not a lawyer, but from my understanding a brief overview follows.

There are four tests that must be applied to a case to determine negligence:

1. The person must be proved to have a **duty of care**.

2. They must be **in breach of that duty**.

3. The negligence must have **caused the harm**.

4. The harm caused must not be **too remote**. I think this broadly means that the harm is something that can be compensated for and sets some limits on the amounts of that compensation.

There are three landmark legal cases that currently set the precedents for where we currently find ourselves in medical defence: Bolam, Bolitho, and Wilsher.

Bolam

This is a case that dates back to 1957 and it is important to consider care in context, not to compare it to the most up-to-date practice in that field. The case radically changed the future of medical law and altered thinking about legal precedents.[4–18]

Mr Bolam was a voluntary patient at an institution and consented to undergo electro-convulsive therapy (ECT). In simple terms, this treatment involves the passage of electricity through the brain and induces a fit. A course of treatment is usually prescribed. It is still used, most commonly for severe depression.

He was not given a muscle relaxant nor restrained. He sustained fractures due to the violent nature of the fits that had been induced.

He tried to claim compensation for:

1. not being given muscle relaxants,

2. not being restrained, and

3. inadequate consent.

I think, to be factually accurate, it was decided by a jury at that time but the law was explained to the jury by the judge. The main question at that time hinged on whether someone else would have done the same. They did not have to prove that the majority of similar doctors would have done the same, simply that someone would have done the same.

This became known as the Bolam test, where if a doctor reaches the standard of a responsible body of medical opinion he/she is not negligent.

Bolitho

In 1997, a baby suffering from breathing difficulties (possibly croup) suffered hypoxic brain damage and eventually died. The nurse called for the doctor to come and see the baby. The doctor did not attend. The doctor claimed that even if they had attended, they would not have intubated the baby. The case seemed to be based on the discussion between differing experts. One group of experts suggested that the baby should have been intubated. A smaller group of experts said they would not have intubated.[18]

The alteration to the law that came about was that you now have to provide the court with 'reasonable and logical' evidence as to why you took that course of action.[18]

Wilsher

In 1988, a premature baby was being cared for on a neonatal intensive care unit and a junior doctor inserted an umbilical artery catheter (UAC). This tube allows regular sampling of blood to look at the oxygen levels. Unfortunately, the tube was placed in a vein by mistake. The junior doctor asked a more senior colleague to review the position on the X-ray which should have alerted them that it was in the wrong vessel. Neither of them identified the mistake.[19]

This case added two new aspects to the law. Firstly, the idea of attributing risk to one of multiple factors and working out the contributions of each. It also highlighted the concept of the comparison of a professional's skills and ability to that of their peer group. The expectations of the junior doctor were that it was a reasonable mistake to make. However, the more senior doctor was expected to have spotted the mistake. This started to bring the levels and quality of supervision under scrutiny.[19]

To sum up the legal bit, you will be judged against whether a reasonable body of your peers would have acted in a similar way at the same point in history (not present-day comparison). You will need to provide reasonable and logical evidence as to why you did it. Supervision levels will also be examined. There must be a duty of care that has been breached. The harm must have been caused by the negligence and the amount of compensation has some limits.[19]

Root cause analysis (RCA)

RCA is a tool that can be used to investigate a serious incident, complaint, or anything that has happened that was less than ideal.

Our current investigation methods within the NHS are variable. They lack the rigour of crash investigation teams in the airline industry. I sometimes ask myself, why? Is it that we only generally kill one at a time? What if no one reports it and we go on making the same mistake? Eventually we could kill as many as there are on an aeroplane. Of course, I know the real answer is, at least in part, due to resources. I believe there are also elements of culture and a better understanding of errors in the airline industry that influence their approach to investigation. It is these two elements within healthcare that I hope to influence.

There is a free RCA toolkit which was originally from the National Patient Safety Agency (<http://www.nrls.npsa.nhs.uk/resources/type/toolkits/?entryid 45=59847>) available to aid with these investigations, as long as the terms and conditions are met (<http://www.nrls.npsa.nhs.uk/resources/rca-conditions/>).

Here is a simplified version of the process for less serious incidents or 'near misses' that incorporates the use of the SHEEP sheet (Figure 2.6).

Having used the term 'near miss' I think it is another term that we need to change. If you nearly miss something, then surely you hit it? Perhaps we should adopt the term a 'nearly event' although 'that was close!' or 'we were lucky!' might be closer to the mark.

Organizational learning

There need to be systems put in place to promote organizational learning and maintain organizational memory. I will discuss the latter first.

Figure 2.6 Nearly event (near miss) investigation.

(10 point plan. Time to complete less than 30 minutes)

1. Nominate a lead (who ideally has had training in group debrief).

2. As soon as possible after the event keep everyone who was involved together (it is much harder to get them back together again later).

3. Ask them all to complete a SHEEP sheet independently. It takes less than 10 minutes. Collect in the SHEEP sheets anonymously.

4. Nominate someone to type as you go along. Not the person leading. Type only a list of actions. Each action should only be documented when indicated by the leader that there is team agreement. Use SMART goals if possible (i.e. Specific Measurable Achievable Realistic and Timely).

5. Run a supportive group debrief, collecting ideas in an open way without blame or finger pointing. Make sure you set some ground rules. Everyone will have chance to speak. No one should interrupt. The finished product of the debrief is to steer the group towards any systems that can be changed to make things safer and any shared learning that has emerged.

6. Agree who will take responsibility for each action and type their name against the action. Remember the time frame. A person who is responsible and a timeframe are the minimum requirement for each action. (Pet hate of mine. Never action someone who is absent. The action is for someone in the room to discuss with the absent person.)

7. Send a joint email to all of those involved *now* with the 'Action Plan' attached. Get everyone to check over your shoulder to make sure you enter all of their email addresses correctly

8. Thank them for being involved.

9. Leader—collate the SHEEP sheets to look for more information that didn't come out in the debrief. Add to the document you have already started if necessary and recirculate.

10. Leader—add SHEEP sheets to database. This way it can be used as a trend analysis tool.

Memory checks

Why do we need them? Unfortunately the human brain is far from perfect. I quite like the analogy that 'it leaks'.

This was a concept to which I was first introduced watching a film. The irony does not escape me when I'm struggling to recall the name of the film. A boy of around 11 ends up on a space ship as the navigator. In fact, that may have featured in the title of the film. Was it The Flight of the Navigator? *An advanced life form had been taking sample life forms from different planets. They had been filling the brains with star charts. They were disappointed to discover that we (humans) only use about 20% of our brains. They also discovered that the human brain leaked!*

The need for a memory check is not only because of the imperfections of the human memory but also because the workforce in any organization is not static. People leave, retire, suffer ill health, go on maternity leave, we employ locums and agency staff, and new staff start regularly. We will perhaps consider ways of helping an individual's memory in a later book.

A system needs to be designed that periodically reminds people of past errors. Whilst an email distribution may be easy for the sender, we have already discussed how that can falsely reassure us that we have disseminated the information and 'communicated'! Like any information flow process, I would suggest a multi-media approach—involve your 'Comms' or Communication department if you have one. Do you even know if you have one?

In addition to the blanket email (if you must), other IT systems (something funky for smart phones, blogs, first page of intranet, screen savers across the institution), consider paper (personalized letters, newsletters, posters (especially inside toilet doors!), in-house magazines, and so on), face to face via the brief/debrief method of Debbie's Diamond and holding patient safety events. There are also the more formal structural roots of line management and governance to explore.

Organizational learning

A system needs to be developed so that there is some central coordination of key messages learnt from errors.

Whilst filling in an incident-reporting electronic form is a step in the right direction, it is only the very first step. The idea of reporting culture is something that intrigues me. It seems to be that people fill in a form as they wish something to change or want to share the learning from their error or problem. There is then an expectation that a miracle will occur and it will all be solved. When you discuss the process with those who receive the forms, my impression is that their expectations are somewhat different. They are expecting the person who fills in the form to make an action plan themselves and implement it.

Somewhat unsurprisingly, this results in a classic case of everyone thinking that somebody else is doing it and therefore nobody does it! This phenomenon has been described as a reporting black hole but I only recently started to understand why it occurs.

The number of reports received centrally are large and unwieldy. The result is that there is over-reliance on the coding system that categorizes the severity of actual or potential harm caused. Only the most serious incidents are explored in any depth.

This is where the SHEEP sheet can help. By filling in the SHEEP sheet when there is an incident, information can be analysed to look for trends. Are the errors in a particular area suggestive of a team problem or something to do with the environment or the equipment? The trends can be looked at in even more detail, right down to individual box frequency. As it is easy to use and analyse the information can be gathered quickly. Only when we can gather the right information can we design the right intervention. The solution is usually system focused.

By using both Debbie's Diamond and all of the dissemination methods mentioned in memory checks, this next step of information sharing is crucial. It is so much less painful to learn from the mistakes of others rather than to have to make them for yourself! We need to generate a learning culture.

Designing the safety intervention needs considerable thought. By adding in another layer of safety (another layer of cheese) remember that you are also lengthening the process and adding complexity. In the current culture of high workload and time pressure, if you increase the length of time above a critical point you will encourage rule breaking and the cutting of corners. There has to be a balance.

Designing an educational intervention also needs a lot of thought. I often hear 'send them on a course!'. It is possible this might help, but it needs to be the right course with the right teaching techniques matched to the preferred learning style of the individual if it is going to have the required impact. There is also a big difference between being 'sent' and choosing to go. Managing expectations prior to attending the educational intervention also plays a key role.

There are other approaches that might be more useful than 'send them on a course!'. Consider coaching, mentoring, clinical psychologist, shadowing, multi-source feedback or 360, appraisal, or occupational health to address individual or team needs.

A more system-based approach might be to highlight opportunities for learning with a patient safety event.

Running a patient safety event

These could be part of monthly governance, a ward or practice meeting, or a more formal organization-wide offering at local or regional level. For me, the latter should be run at least annually. These events should be multi-professional, aiming to be yet another moment to bring down the silos of 'us' and 'them' culture. I refer to the differences between clinical and non-clinical and between the different clinical professions. There should also be mixing of all grades to try and reduce some of the steep hierarchy that exists. There should be an emphasis on 'we' are all working towards the same goal.

These should be designed to appeal to all learning styles. Whilst PowerPoint presentations may appeal to the theorists, they do little for some of the other adult learners. The few hours or half day or day should include something for everyone. A well-known, engaging speaker will help to raise the profile of the event and may serve as the first 'carrot' to encourage participation.

It is worth considering whether to make it an event where staff can showcase and celebrate their success too. Posters and oral presentations, perhaps with the added incentive of other carrots (prizes or simply a reward for entering), may further encourage interest in the event. Caution: the prizes and rewards are now more tightly controlled and should be in some way related to the topic of the day. A colleague purchased a number of safety-related books and gave one to each of the participants who submitted a presentation.

The activists and pragmatists (broad generalization) are better if there is some-thing to do. By rotating them through a series of workshops in smaller groups with interactive tasks in each workshop, you will generally stimulate them more than with a didactic approach (i.e. talking at them).

Some of the more difficult groups sometimes respond well to something we have nicknamed 'competitive problem solving'. Divide the group into teams and ask them to come up with solutions to a complex problem. Ideally some-thing with which you genuinely do need some help. Frame it that no one has previously solved this issue and you need their combined expertise to come up with a creative solution. Try to use humour and keep it fun and light-hearted.

Board and executive engagement are an essential component if that is relevant to your organizational structure. Otherwise, consider who your stakeholders might be. Who holds the purse strings? Who has the final say in change and influence in your organization?

The organization should also be considered on many levels. For example, there should be learning at the micro-climate level of the ward, through other wards across a Trust, across the region, and then nationally and internationally. Within healthcare we need to start thinking about this level of large-scale learning and how we going to create systems to tackle it.

Engagement with people and encouraging them to take ownership of the changes that are required to produce organizational learning is the way to pitch it. I would steer clear of didactic, blame, or anything that could be construed as preaching. A tailor-made solution designed by the people in the area where the problem is will result in a sustained change if well supported. There is a completely different response if people feel something is being imposed on them. I believe this coaching approach is vital when introducing any improvement model.

There are elements of a human factors approach that link in with the newer trends of health quality improvement (QI). The ideas underlying the latter include the principles of reducing variation by increased standardization, reducing harm, decreasing error, removing duplication, and minimizing waste. In addition to QI methodology, the theories around Lean and Six Sigma and the Productive Series (ward, theatre, and general practice) are all worth exploring.

The systems that are associated with the environment and equipment will be discussed in the chapters with those headings.

Key points from Chapters 1 and 2

- To err is human.

- We need to embed an open culture. Culture is one of many informal systems in which we function.

- There should be an inquisitive approach to error that seeks out the learning and shares it: the learning culture.

- This should include 'memory checks' and 'safety events'.

- The new error checklist—the SHEEP sheet—helps gather more information following an actual event or a nearly event. It is quick and easy to use.

- There is a simple 10-point plan for analysis of a nearly event.

- The SHEEP sheet can be used for trend analysis.

- Information flow across an organization can be achieved using a brief/debrief model using Debbie's Diamond. This should be a patient-centric approach using the simple format from Table 2.2.

- We need to raise the standards for writing of SOPs. A simple set of minimum criteria is suggested in Box 2.1.

- Things are not always what they seem: avoid assumption.

- 'What am I missing here?' is a healthy question to keep asking.

- Systems errors are commonly part of the holes in the Swiss cheese and should feature in the solutions for improved safety.

References

1. Pascal B. *Lettres provinciales*, 1656/1657.
2. Gawande A. The checklist: if something so simple can transform intensive care, what else can it do? *New Yorker* 2007;10 December:86–101.
3. Gawande A. Checklists for success inside the OR and beyond: an interview with Atul Gawanda, MD, FACS. Interview by Tony Peregrin. *Bulletin of the American College of Surgeons* 2010;95(5):24–7.
4. Badenoch J. Brushes with Bolam. Where will it lead? *Medico-Legal Journal* 2004;72(Pt 4):127–42.
5. Brahams D. Superspecialists and the Bolam test. *Lancet* 1995;345(8949):575.
6. Brahams D. 'Super-specialists' and the Bolam test. *Medico-Legal Journal* 1995;63 (Pt 1):4–5.
7. Burdon J. From Bolam to Ipp: an examination of the standard of care in medical negligence cases since 1957. *Internal Medicine Journal* 2004;34(12):662.
8. Feenan DK. Beyond Bolam: responding to the patient. *Medical Law International* 1994;1(2):177–93.
9. Fenwick P, Beran RG. Informed consent—should Bolam be rejected? *Medicine and Law* 1997;16(2):215–23.
10. Harpwood V. Medical negligence: a chink in the armour of the Bolam test? *Medico-Legal Journal* 1996;64 (Pt 4):179–85.
11. Hourigan KJ. From Bolam to Ipp. *Internal Medicine Journal* 2005;35(7):438–9; author reply 39–40.
12. Jones JW. The healthcare professional and the Bolam test. *British Dental Journal* 2000;188(5):237–40.
13. Kirby M. Patients' rights—why the Australian courts have rejected 'Bolam'. *Journal of Medical Ethics* 1995;21(1):5–8.
14. Reynard J, Marsh H. The development of consent from Bolam to Chester: what you need to know and what your patients are entitled to know. *BJU International* 2009;103(11):1458–61.
15. Samanta A, Mello MM, Foster C, Tingle J, Samanta J. The role of clinical guidelines in medical negligence litigation: a shift from the Bolam standard? *Medical Law Review* 2006;14(3):321–66.
16. Samanta A, Samanta J. Legal standard of care: a shift from the traditional Bolam test. *Clinical Medicine* 2003;3(5):443–6.
17. Shanmugam K. Testing the Bolam Test: consequences of recent developments. *Singapore Medical Journal* 2002;43(1):7–11.
18. Sooriakumaran P. The changing face of medical negligence law: from Bolam to Bolitho. *British Journal of Hospital Medicine* 2008;69(6):335–8.
19. Brahams D. The Wilsher case. *Medico-Legal Journal* 1988;56 (Pt 2):49–51.

3

The 'H' of SHEEP: Human interaction

Knowledge comes, but wisdom lingers

Lord Alfred Tennyson
Locksley Hall (1842), line 141

Introduction

Let's start by exploring the 'H' of the algorithm (see Figure 3.1).

We will divide this topic up to look at team working, task-related issues, and then hone down to particular behaviours. Communication, by which I mean face-to-face interaction, will be given a dedicated chapter all of its own.

For me, and our early research reinforces my gut feeling, this area of human interaction is where the heart of many of our problems lie in healthcare. I've spent a lot of time reflecting on why I think this is the case and I have two answers.

The primary answer is that central to everything we do is a human being—the patient. This is unlike any other high-reliability organization that we are told we should try and emulate. The majority of those seem to surround an inanimate object, be it an aeroplane or a nuclear reactor or a train or a space shuttle or an oil rig. I admit that we can learn good lessons from all of these but none has the central aspect to everything they do with such variability. Each human being has such a high degree of complexity and each one is unique. There are the standard gender differences, differences associated with race, ongoing physiological changes from fetus to neonate through paediatric years and adolescence to adulthood, and then begins the wonderful ageing process. I have yet to add in anatomical anomalies, disease states, and pathology. On top of that there are the emotional, psychological, and cognitive aspects of the individual and then the added interactions with loved ones and relatives. There is no other industry that faces that degree of central complexity and variability.

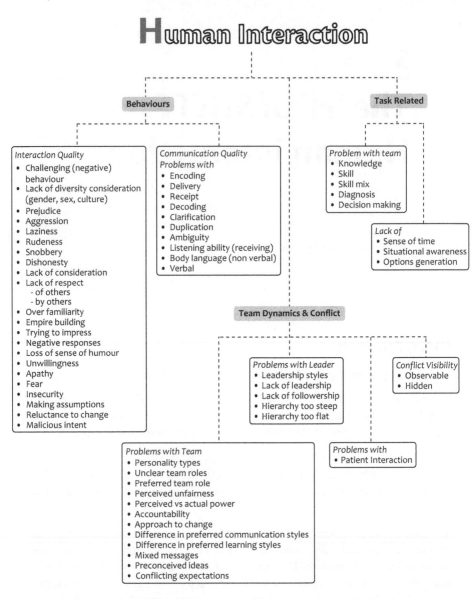

Figure 3.1 'H'—the SHEEP model.

The second reason is that not only is everything with do revolving around the central figure—the patient,a human interaction in itself—but we often work in large, changing teams. The large size and their unstable nature both play a part. There are huge differences in what might constitute a team across the different areas of healthcare.

If we begin in primary care there might be a practice manager, receptionists, nurses, and GPs plus or minus pharmacists and a few others. The core team may well be fairly static barring sickness, maternity leave, and retirements in the most part. The size of the team is fairly controlled. A number of those individuals will be in post for a large number of years. If working well, the team will begin to learn its strengths and weaknesses including the subtle nuances of personality types and preferred ways of working. It will have time to evolve and grow together over time. There are real benefits in investing in growing this team. We will think about how best to go about this shortly. Before we do that the first step is to identify who is in your team(s).

Consider for a moment the team that you work in. If you have time grab a piece of paper and a pen and try Exercise 3.1.

Exercise 3.1 Circles of influence

1.	Take a moment to imagine yourself at work. Are all of your days the same? Divide the paper up to represent the different days, but group the same days together. For example, theatre days, clinic days, ward days, and office days rather than days of the week.
2.	Put yourself in the centre of each type of day. (Represent yourself however you like—a circle, a square, a stickman?)
3.	Now consider the people you work with. I will ask you to draw them, too, in a minute. Do you work with different people on different days? How much influence do they have on you and you on them? How much time do you spend with them?
4.	With you as the central figure I want you to draw in the other people. If you spend more time with them, they have more influence on you or you have a lot of influence on them, draw them closer to you. If you spend only a small amount of time with them or the influence levels are lower, then draw them further away from you. You can put a line between yourself and them to create a 'spokes of a bicycle wheel' look if you wish.
5.	Repeat the exercise for each of teams that you work with.
6.	Sit back and have a look at it. How many teams are you working in? Are the teams the same each week or do they vary? Which are the best of those teams? Why is that? What makes it good? Are there any dysfunctional teams amongst them? What is your role in that team? Could you help to move the team forward?
7.	Hold onto this for now, we will return to it when we have learnt a bit more.

Michael West[1] points out the detrimental affects of working in pseudo-teams and yet within secondary care, these abound. Have a look at your teams, are they true teams that work together regularly or is rather more random than that? Building a stable team can lower stress levels and encourage staff retention.

I think it is helpful to consider the two situations of stable teams versus variable teams slightly separately.

The unstable/constantly changing/ dynamic team

Even within this concept there may be differences depending on where you work. Some of you will work a shift pattern where the staff that you work with will be drawn from a large pool. You will know some of them well and others more casually. An example is a ward of nursing staff that are rotated to work shifts. Depending on the off duty, they will work with different people on different days but they will generally know most of the other ward staff.

There will be other times when very few people involved have even met each other. They find themselves suddenly together often because of a task that has arisen. An example of this would be a cardiac arrest team. A number of people of different grades carry the cardiac arrest bleep but it is a fairly random distribution of different rotas at different grades and across different specialties. There are more possible variations of people who won't know each other at all. They arrive at a bedside in an emergency setting to perform a task for a designated amount of time until the task has reached a resolution and then they return to their other roles.

The team in the latter has little time to establish itself but if it is to function effectively, it must gel together quickly. Here are a few tips to help with this eventuality.

CRM originally referred to Crew Resource Management within the airline industry. As healthcare progressed the acronym was adapted to represent Crisis Resource Management. The example in Box 3.1 shows how it was adapted by David Gaba[2-4] into anaesthetic crisis resource management (ACRM). A whole family of this type of crisis resource management now exists.[5,6]

This original list has been modified over time and multiple variations exist. Another example is included in Box 3.2.

I will develop these lists further subsequently, as for me, they don't go far enough.

From these beginnings several other layers of tools have developed to use to assess non-technical skills. There are generic NOTECH (non-technical) skills that were originally taken from the airline industry and then were adapted to healthcare.[8,9] I have developed my own debriefing prompt based on this, G-NO-TECS.

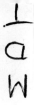

Box 3.1   Key points of ACRM[7]

Points regarding decision-making and cognition

- Know the environment

- Anticipate and plan

- Use all available information and cross check

- Prevent or manage fixation errors

- Use cognitive aids.

Points regarding teamwork and resource management

- Exercise leadership and followership

- Call for help early

- Communicate effectively

- Distribute the workload

- Mobilize all available resources for optimum management.

Source: David M. Gaba et al., Simulation-Based Training in Anesthesia Crisis Resource Management (ACRM): A Decade of Experience, *Simulation and Gaming*, Volume 32, issue, 2, pp. 175–193, Copyright © 2001 Sage Publications, Inc. Reprinted by permission of SAGE Publications.

Box 3.2   Variation CRM

Team

1. Anticipation/planning

2. Communication

3. Leadership/assertiveness

4. Awareness and utilization of all available resources

5. Distribution of workload and mobilization of help

6. Routine re-evaluation of situation

7. Awareness and utilization of all available information.

For use in the Emergency Department

8. Triage/prioritization

9. Efficient management of multiple patients

10. Effective coping with disruptions/distractions.

Individual

11. Call for help early.

There are also more specific tools for different specialties, developed by Rhona Flin and others.[10–17] These include ANTS for anaesthetists, NOTSS for surgeons, SPLINTS for scrub nurses, and tools for ophthalmology, psychiatry, obstetrics, and histopathology with more being developed all the time. Another soapbox moment is included in Box 3.3.

Box 3.3 Warning—another soapbox moment!

I have quite strong ideas about how these tools should and more importantly should **not** be used. This has to do with the differences between summative and formative assessment, I think the former has no place in non-technical skills. *I realize this momentary lapse into education speak will have an interesting affect on some of you. Pause. Were you one of the ones who just rolled their eyes? If you were, then bear with me while I explain.*

If you have passed through the British education system then you will be very familiar with summative assessment, even if you didn't know it. In the broadest of terms it means reaching an arbitrary level—be it pass/fail or to obtain an A, B, or C. There is some sort of test or hurdle to quantify your achievement and perhaps make an inference that you are ready for the next level, whatever that might mean. On the other hand you could say that for a doctor taking an exam where the pass mark is 75%, that they don't know 25% of the information! Scary but true.

So, why am I so against measuring people's non-technical skill performance? Why don't I think it is helpful to assess their behaviour on one scenario on one particular day and make inferences about the whole of the practice? Why don't I think that telling someone they are 3 out of 4 on one particular skill, and 2 out of 4 on another, on a particular day in a particular scenario is helpful for them? Have a think for a minute. How will it make them feel? How will it affect their learning, knowing you are measuring them? Will it alter what you are measuring if you know it is being measured?

I am not alone with my soapbox about summative assessment. If you have time, find Donald Clark and his TED lecture on YouTube.

Have you discovered the TED series? I find them inspirational. They are a group of creatively funded lectures from speakers who are world renowned in their field. They speak on all subjects, life and the universe included. Anyone who can make statistics not just interesting but exciting needs a medal in my book! They are free to watch on the Internet.

Box 3.4 Challenge and rapport

I think it is useful here to consider a parallel with coaching and 'facilitating'. (I deliberately do not use the words 'teaching' nor 'instructing' at this point, as they are different.) I would like to introduce some ideas around challenge and rapport and illustrate some analogies with learning and trust.

So what does the term 'challenge' mean for you? This is a useful concept to explore when coaching or facilitating. It is useful to discover what it looks like when you observe it.

For me, it is about being pushed. How hard do I feel I'm being pushed relative to my comfort zone?

When we are leading in a coaching style or facilitating, the better we know them and the more comfortable someone is with us, the harder they will be able to be pushed whilst they still feel safe. (This fits with the challenge and rapport model which is worth looking up if you fancy exploring this in a bit more depth.)

Put quite simply then, if you get to know someone and they know you, you can push then a bit harder. You want them to be in the zone of awareness but not out of their comfort zone. If you can manage it, to work them near the edge of the comfort zone will achieve the greatest results but takes skill and practice.

> For the clinicians who remember their Starling curve, I would like to offer another analogy. If instead of the filling of the heart, you imagine a learning curve. You want the learner to be engaged and not bored so they require a certain amount of stimulation but you don't want to push them too far. If their stress levels rise above a certain point they stop learning. (This is what I call the bunny-in-the-headlights moment.) Each of your learners has their own curve in every different situation. The only ways to know where they are to observe them and look for clues in their non-verbal communication and behaviour or to ask them.

Now let's return to the questions.

> *How will it affect their learning, knowing you are measuring them?*

> *Will it alter what you are measuring if you know it is being measured?*

In my experience the measurement does indeed affect the behaviour. I have also found that it inhibits learning. I would like to propose that we stop trying to quantify behaviour. It is a continuum. The cut-off points between an arbitrary 2 out of 4 and 3 out of 4 are grey and are open to observer bias and interpretation. Whilst I admit that the tools have been validated, this approach is not for me. I find a much more helpful approach is a debriefing/coaching style conversation. See Box 3.4 for an introduction to the Challenge and Rapport model.

Generic Non–Technical Skills G–NO–TECS Debrief Prompt	COMMENTS

Team
• Leadership skills (including approachability of leader)
• Followership skills (including assertiveness of followers)
• Team building and maintaining (including hierarchy management)
    o Clear and appropriate role allocation
    o Consideration and support of others
• Conflict solving	

Decision-Making • Problem definition and diagnosis (commentating, generating shared mental model) • Option generation (encouraging team input, avoiding fixation error) • Risk assessment and option selection • Regular review of decision as new information emerges	
Tasks • Providing and maintaining standards • Workload management (including distraction management and prioritization of tasks) • Knowledge of and ability to use equipment	
Awareness – Situational • Awareness of the systems • Awareness of the environment • Awareness of time (use of time checks) • Ability to plan ahead (anticipate need for staff/equipment/change of environment) • Maintenance of care, compassion and dignity **Awareness – Self** • Stress, fatigue, cognitive workload, time pressure, call for help if appropriate • Balcony and dance floor, Swan	
Information Management • Gathering of information (from patient, relatives, team, other teams, records) • Sharing of information (including use of structured handover tool e.g. SBAR) • Use of cognitive aids (guidelines, BNF, internet) • Listening, non-verbal and verbal communication • Read back, active identification, cross check, opening questions, avoidance of pronouns	

Figure 3.2 The abbreviated G-NO-TECS tool with the headings only. Full version in appendix 2.

Please don't get me wrong, I love the G-NO-TECs tools as a framework for a conversation. I think they are the gold standard to help encourage a group-led debrief around non-technical skills (where, ideally, I do little except keep a gentle hand on the rudder). In fact, I think they should be used routinely as part of every simulation and perhaps one day, when daily debrief happens at the end of every shift/day, within all of our daily team working? (Alright, I admit it, this is a bit of an end of the rainbow moment for me, but a girl can dream!)

In Figure 3.2 and Appendix 2 is an example of my completely generic G-NO-TECs debriefing prompt.

So let's have a look at each of those sections in more detail.

Team working

How are you going to build a good team? What does a good team look like? How will you know when you are in one?

Team building and maintaining

Each team member needs to have a clear role that is appropriate and will make them feel valued. There must be respectful interaction where everyone feels able to contribute and that they are listened to. There should be ample opportunities to express an opinion while the other members of the team listen actively. There should be clarification and checking of the meaning. There should be no judgement nor should there be criticism but it should be a safe enough environment to deliver respectful feedback. There should be praise. The members should be approachable. They need to be united around a common goal and have a shared understanding of what they are trying to achieve.

Support and consideration of others

There is no place for a 'mood hoover' on my team.

I want you to think about the phrase 'mood hoover'. Do you know what it is? I want you to imagine a time when everyone was quite happily getting on with things until an individual arrived and sucked the enthusiasm and happiness from the room. We can all have an off day but it is not acceptable to become a repeat offender.

I would much rather have optimists on my team. When we move to look at stable teams we will look at choosing people to fit together but in an unstable/dynamic team we don't have that luxury, we are often just thrown together by circumstances and expected to cope.

The team needs to support each other. It needs to be aware of what others are doing and how they are coping. It needs to be aware of who is overstretched or at the edge of their comfort zone and who might have spare capacity. There needs to be constant vigilance and regular review of how each member is doing in their role and adjustment accordingly. Each member needs to feel supported and that they can be honest about how they are coping.

This should not include the attitude which was abundant when I first trained which was 'feel free to cope!'.

Conflict resolution

Whilst conflict may arise within the group, there should be a clear way for it to be dealt with that aims at win–win outcomes or collaboration with an equal amount of compromise. We will return to conflict resolution later but remember it can be positive and perhaps even essential to have differing opinions expressed, as long as it is all handled respectfully.

Team spirit

For me, there is also something about the spirit of the team. It is difficult to capture in words. Perhaps it is a sense of fun or optimism that will see you through a challenge, no matter how hard it might seem right now. Perhaps there is a sense of real belief and trust in everyone to pull together and give it their all. Perhaps there is some feeling of the what 'we British refer to as spirit of the Blitz'. I suspect this is quite an individual thing. What would you like your team spirit to be? How will you go about generating it?

Decision-making

In an emergency or urgent clinical setting it is important to gather information quickly from all available sources, weigh it up, and make a plan. The plan may be reliant on forming a provisional diagnosis that will need to be reviewed regularly as new information is received and as the situation is ongoing. The plan needs to be clearly formed with agreement from the team, so that there is a shared understanding of what they are trying to achieve. The team should all be able to challenge the plan with new ideas of alternative courses of action and any new information. There should be someone with responsibility for the decisions but this person may change. There should be regular review of the diagnosis and the plan and the progress to date. Resources of prepared plans that suit the situation should be sort.

For those of you who like mnemonics:

Diagnosis
Option generation

Decide
Assessment
Review.

The way information is gathered will be influenced by the urgency of the situation.

Information gathering in a clinical emergency/crisis

I realize that not everyone works in an emergency clinical setting so if that's you, you can either skip this bit or use it for a bit of empathy for your colleagues that do or look for any learning that you can extract from it that may have some relevance to you. It is too important for me to brush over though.

In an absolute emergency (imminent or already in cardiac arrest) then the ABCDE approach of advanced life support comes into play. (A for airway, B for breathing, C for cardiovascular meaning the heart and blood that it pumps around the body, D for dysfunction which in broad terms means conscious level, and E for exposure to encourage you to look at the whole patient and consider them in their entirety.) This is a **S**ystem.

The system allows for information gathering in a predefined way and initiates the management of each of those matching parts of the body at the same time. There is a coupled approach of information gathering and making a decision.

Is the airway OK?
If no, what shall we do to fix it? Do something. Reassess. Is airway ok now?
If yes, move to B.
Is B ok?
If no, what shall we do to fix it? Do something. Reassess. Is B ok now?
If yes, move to C.
And so on.

By dividing the team up so that each member has clear roles it is possible for multiple processes to happen simultaneously. This role allocation should be confirmed out loud and ideally with sharing of names. The role needs to be appropriate to the level of experience of the individual.

People

1. Named person for Airway and Breathing.

2. Named person for Cardiovascular and IV access (putting in a drip so that it is possible to take a blood test, give drugs and give fluids) and giving cardiac massage if required.

3. Named person for fetching crash trolley and getting monitoring on, using defibrillator if required, and giving drugs.

4. Named person to do the timing and write things down, may prepare drugs for giving when they are due.

5. Named person to lead the team (ideally doing no technical tasks), free to: commentate (talks out loud through thought processes and plans), information gather, facilitate decision-making, control distractions, monitor workload and progress, review regularly, anticipate and plan, make decisions.

6. Named person to call for more help, fetch resources as needed (ideally as anticipated by leader or others ahead of time), locate algorithm, and help any team member who might need support.

Process

1. ABCDE is initiated and roles are decided as listed earlier. Decisions in this setting are, therefore, layered. Responsibility for decision-making in each subtask is ideally delegated to each individual. Each individual gives progress reports to the leader. The leader has the big picture and can hopefully gather information from each person in turn and start to build up an overview. A working diagnosis may be formed. This may be as broad as verbalizing, 'This is an anaesthetic emergency!' or 'This is a cardiac arrest!'.

2. Life-saving actions are underway to assess and support ABCDE in the team formation. Each member of the team has a clear role, appropriate for their ability. Call for help early if senior help or just more pairs of hands required.

3. Options are generated. A good team leader should ask opening up questions that encourage the team to give their ideas:

   'Any thoughts on what this might be?'

   'What are we missing here?'

   'What else could this be?'

4. Ideally the team leader will now decide on a diagnosis and verbalize this diagnosis so that the team has a shared understanding of the problem. I purposefully have put the diagnosis stage after the option generation phase. I find if the team leader says, 'This is x, isn't it?' then the team will simply agree with the leader. There is more chance of fixation error.

5. Locate and use the appropriate algorithm for the situation. Have it clearly displayed for the team leader and time keeper at the very least. Share which algorithm you are using with the team.

6. Initial management is now underway and the patient is having life-supporting treatment. More information gathering and assessment can now take place.

   Our team need to gather the '**history**'. This involves locating a number of different types of resources including any of the following:

   ◆ Notes, blood results, x-rays, GP letters

   ◆ Information from the patients nurse

   ◆ Information from the patient's medical team

   ◆ Information from anyone who witnessed the event who was first on the scene

   ◆ Information from paramedics if they are being brought in from home

   ◆ Information from relatives.

7. Ensure communication includes clarification/read back/cross checking (see Chapter 7).

8. Reassess the patient at a frequency that is either suggested in the algorithm or every few minutes. This means a full ABCDE type assessment.

   Team leader says, 'OK, let's review the patient from the top starting with **A**—How is the airway?' Airway person answers about whether the airway is secure and which device they are using, and whether there are any issues. A subplan for **A** is put in place.

   Team leader says, '**B**?' The chest is re-examined by observing chest movement and listening with a stethoscope. Use information from any relevant monitoring (Saturation reading if available (not in a full cardiac arrest!) and end-tidal CO2) or blood results (e.g. blood gases) are considered. Decide on a subplan for **B**.

   Team leader says, 'Moving on to **C**?' Examination of the patient's cardiovascular status and gathering of any relevant information from the monitoring takes place (including blood pressure, rate, rhythm, perfusion, capillary refill, volume status, electrical activity—again some of these are not relevant to full arrest). A subplan for **C** is decided.

   Team leader asks for an assessment of **D**. This includes an assessment of conscious level perhaps using one of two **S**ystems either:

   a. AVPU[18] which stands for **a**lert, responding to **v**oice, responding to **p**ain or **u**nresponsive

   OR

    b.   Glasgow Coma Score[19] if appropriate.

Any other neurological assessment that may be relevant and a blood glucose level are also checked at this juncture. Any relevant subplan for **D** is formulated.

E. The team leader encourages an examination of the whole patient, looking for any other clues with the examination, monitoring and test results. A temperature is also relevant at this stage. If there is action to be taken for **E**, a subplan is initiated.

9. It is useful for the team leader to verbalize a summary of all the findings. At this point the working diagnosis is presented along with which algorithm is being used.

10. Repeat option generation as per number 2, i.e.:

    'Any thoughts on what else this might be?'

    'What are we missing here?'

    'What else could this be?'

11. Is more help needed? (Either for senior advice or just more pairs of hands.)

12. Are there any more cognitive aids to consider? (Internet/guidelines.)

13. Anticipating the next few steps, is there anything else or anyone else needed?

14. Team leader should share the next steps with team and ask them if they have any other ideas? Or is anything missing?

15. Return to number 5 and repeat stages 5–13.

Leadership

Leadership will be discussed in many guises at different stages of this book and more extensively in the next book. For now, we are specifically considering the leadership role in an emergency scenario which will often be in an unstable/unfamiliar/dynamic team setting.

There needs to be a conversation about who is going to lead. If you arrive at an emergency setting and it isn't obvious who is leading or whether anyone is leading, then the question needs to be asked. A simple, 'Who is leading?' should suffice.

There are various options for deciding on the most suitable person to lead. It shouldn't just default to the more senior person in the room. This may be the best person to lead, but it may be that their skills are best employed to perform a particular task.

The hierarchy system in secondary care is quite fascinating and it exists within professions and between them. It seems to vary in different specialties. The more traditional amongst you may be wondering what is so bad about this ingrained behaviour. Whilst a directive or old school heroic leader may be seen as a strong decision-maker there is a problem with this approach.

There have now been some very serious errors in which this steep hierarchy (also known as large power distance) has played a part. There was a case of wrong-site surgery where a junior member of the team tried to challenge the consultant about the side at the beginning of the case. The junior member was told to 'pipe down' as the consultant had lots of years of experience and what did they know by comparison? Unfortunately, the wrong-site surgery proceeded and the working kidney was removed. Steep hierarchy inhibiting challenge was also a key factor in the case of Elaine Bromiley.[20] In this case the nursing staff knew what needed to happen but they felt unable to broach the subject with the consultants. They gently tried to encourage a different course of action by wheeling in some equipment for they lacked the assertiveness skills that were required and the consultants lacked the skills to empower them to put forward their ideas and be heard.

If you are a leader, I would like you to pause and think:

◆ How can you make sure you are an approachable leader?

◆ How would you make sure your team feel able to put forward their ideas?

◆ How can you ensure that a junior member of your team would be able to challenge you if you were making a mistake?

I am really hoping that no one who is reading this is still under the illusion that they are so good that mistakes are things that can only happen to someone else? If that is you, you are my biggest worry of all!

I have interestingly heard it expressed that the problem is not with the approach-ability of the leaders but with the assertiveness of the followers. I sighed. Whilst I agree that if you see someone making a mistake, you have a responsibility to keep on expressing your opinion as you are the patient's advocate. The junior members of the team are unlikely to be able to bring about culture change on their own. I believe it is those of us who lead who need to role model good behaviour.

An example of this type of leadership was listed earlier, where the leader regularly asks the team, 'What am I missing?'. This approach is multifaceted. As well as genuinely hoping to use the 'many heads are better than one' approach, it also admits the vulnerability of the leader (no leader is all-knowing) and could be missing something. This approach also helps to build a team where everyone's opinion is valued and actually the leader feels more supported.

Also take care when there are several people of the same grade who could all be leading. This case of flat hierarchy can also cause problems as no one makes the decisions. In this case, there needs to be a thorough conversation about each person's role. Establish if anyone has a particular practical skill that is required—if it is a difficult task, let the most experienced practically do the task. Let the other one stand back and keep the big picture and lead.

We are aiming for 15 degrees of hierarchy, i.e. not flat and not steep

The leader needs to keep an eye on all of the various team activities. They will help form the various subplans for managing each system and monitoring of progress against each of these subgoals. They will also be watching the overall aims and goals and the progress with each of these against the algorithm or guideline or plan. There is also a quality control element of this role (e.g. the rate and depth of cardiac compressions during cardiac massage). It is important how this quality control is communicated though. Try asking questions. In the example given you could enquire, 'What rate are you aiming for?'. If they know the answer then, following affirmation and praise if appropriate and not conde-scending, you have the option to open a conversation about going a little faster. If they don't know, you can educate them and then encourage them to up the tempo.

We will discuss a detrimental leadership style called 'pace setting' later. It is important not to fall into that mode.

The leader as we have said helps with each subplan for each system as well as the overall plan. They also help the team to anticipate what personnel and equipment may be required in the future and start to plan how to mobilize it. There might be a necessity to move venue (e.g. to go to CT scan or to theatre or to another hospital all together). The transport, equipment, and personnel will all need to be planned carefully. There will need to be exten-sive communication with the current team and perhaps with a number of other teams.

Whilst all of these other tasks are in play, the leader needs to monitor the work-load (both cognitive and task) of each of the team members and themselves. It may be necessary to support an inexperienced team member or substitute someone who is tired during cardiac massage or notice that someone is getting stressed. It may be necessary to call for help for more experience or more pairs of hands. All of these things must be juggled by the leader, hopefully with sup-portive input from the team who are empowered to offer up their suggestions in an orderly and respectful way. They are not talking over each other and they are all listening.

Situational awareness

Awareness of the passage of time

It is incredibly easy to lose track of time in an emergency setting. People become so focused on the task that they just simply lose track of time.

How long is it that they have been trying to establish intravenous access (put in a drip)? How long have they been trying to intubate (put a tube into a trachea or windpipe)? There are clear guidelines on each of these activities, so what is it that makes us persist?

◆ Is it that we have done that task many times before, so we know if we try long enough we will get there?

◆ Is it that we nearly did it that time, so if we have just one more go maybe we will get there?

◆ Is it a fear of failure? Or that failure is not an option because the patient needs it *now*?

◆ Is it that our cone of focus just becomes so narrow that we block out our surroundings and focus on the success of the task, forsaking everything else?

◆ Are there times when that degree of focus has been advantageous in the past? (Personal examples include a range from childhood in a school class-room when I refuse to be interrupted by a disruptive child on the other side of the room to as an adult, trying to write a paper for a deadline when my own children are playing nearby.)

◆ Is there an element of complacency involved?

◆ Is arrogance a contributory factor?

◆ Is it a complex mix of any of these points and it is different in each situation?

What is more important is how are we going to stop it happening to us?

We mentioned already that if you have a big enough team then it becomes one person's role to time keep and document. It is a vital role. The person taking this role needs to give verbal time checks throughout the progress of the incident. In addition there may be specific tasks that are time critical.

Example of time-critical task

We are taught that we should intubate in less than 30 seconds and that if we cannot achieve it in that time then we should stop and continue to squeeze a bag so that we can blow oxygen into the patient's lungs. We are taught that we should ask someone to time us or count for us while we perform this task. When someone is intubating in a routine manner only they can see inside the patient's mouth. Only they can see whether it is an easy one or a difficult one. I teach my juniors to talk out loud as they perform the task. This **S**ystem of 'commentating' has several functions. It slows the trainee down and makes the step of looking for the anatomical landmarks more definite. This should help them stay calmer and feel more in control. It allows all the other members of the team (the person who is assisting them and the supervisor if there is one) to know what stage they are at and to have a shared understanding of how difficult the task is at that stage.

When they have obtained a view of the vocal cords there is a grading **S**ystem which I also ask them to verbalize. This tells the person they are working with whether it is all going to be straightforward or whether it will be necessary to find more equipment to make the task easier. Once the tube is in there is another **S**ystem to confirm it is in the right place (Box 3.5). I find the system is rarely used in its entirety and I often ask myself why is it that corners are cut?

◆ Is it the 'it won't happen to me culture'?

◆ I've been doing this for years?

◆ Time pressure?

◆ It's over the top? The process is too long winded? It's not necessary?

. . . and yet people still die from the tube not being in the right place.

Box 3.5

Just in case you were wondering about confirming tube placement—for me, the gold standard should be along the lines of verbalizing information illustrated in the example that follows:

◆ 'Grade 1 view, I've seen the tube go between the cords.'

◆ '20 cm at the lips.'

◆ 'Misting.'

◆ Count bagging 1, 2, 3, 4, 5, 6 and count 'CO_2 breaths 1, 2, 3, 4, 5, 6' out loud.

◆ Listen to both axillae and over the stomach with a good old-fashioned stethoscope, 'yes air entry, yes air entry, no sounds. Happy to tie it in'.

Of course, this is a standard for now, on the day that I'm writing, but may be improved upon in the future with new developments.

Awareness of systems

I have tried to slip in examples of Systems as we went along. I have included a system for dividing up roles, a system of assessing the patient and initiating management, a system for non-technical skills (G-NO-TECs), a system for crisis resource management, a system for assessing conscious level, a system to check for correct tube placement, etc.

Which system is being used needs to be verbalized within the team so that there is a shared understanding of the plan. Regular review of whether the right systems are being used needs to be built in and an opportunity to offer up new ideas enabled. Quality control is also a system.

There should be a conversation about whether there are cognitive aids for this situation. If it is not clear whether an algorithm is being used ask, 'Which algorithm are we using?' or 'Is there a guideline for this?', 'Where can I find it?'. Don't be put off by someone appearing to know the guideline; it might still be useful to have it handy. In times of stress our memory is not as reliable.

Awareness of the external environment

Whilst the weather may be very relevant to a pilot or a sailor, it is generally of less interest to those of us healthcare when we are managing a patient. Of course, snow and ice have health implications and there may be times when transferring between hospitals we may need to consider the conditions. In broad terms though this is not the external environment we are referring to.

We may need to be aware of the workload within our department and how our actions with one patient may have implications of resources for others. There may be interruptions that need to be controlled or delegated. There may be a changing list of priorities as a patient elsewhere deteriorates.

We may need to consider the whereabouts of senior cover who may not be on site and anticipate the need for them to travel.

We may need to mobilize equipment from elsewhere in the hospital and we need to find someone to find it, move it, and allow time for it to arrive.

We may need to move the patient. This needs to be carefully planned.

Do you have a system and a checklist for every time you do this? Have you checked that you have the right equipment, drugs, and personnel to cover different eventualities? Do you have a backup if something fails? What if you get stuck in the lift? Will the bed fit through the space in the corridor and then through the doors to the CT scanner or do you need to be on a special trolley? Is the receiving team ready for you? Do they know what your expectations are and therefore what equipment they might need? Have you completed an ABCDE assessment just prior to leaving? Is there time pressure? Has this been shared with all teams to ensure a shared understanding? Have you remembered all the notes, blood results, and relevant tests results? Do you know where you are going and how to get there? Have you got to cancel something for another patient as this one is now an emergency? Have that patient and their team been informed?

Knowing your environment can be very important when you need to find something in a hurry. Standardization of clinical areas can help with this and systems to facilitate this are covered in the Environment chapter (Chapter 4).

All of the earlier points have been based on a variable team that is almost 'thrown together' because of circumstance. They have an emergency, shared focus but they are time poor and they may not work together again in that particular grouping.

We need to consider the contrasting team which is stable and long term. Of course, there will be a spectrum in between.

Team building for the long term

Many of us don't get to choose the team that we work in but over time we may get to influence its make up or the way that it works.

I'm going to start by introducing a few mainstream tools. No single tool is a holy grail to producing a happy, efficient well-motivated team but each tool may add a little more insight into the interactions between the people involved. I believe that if each member becomes more self-aware, the team can look for strengths and gaps and identify where there might be 'rubs'.

Let's start with an old faithful—the Myers Briggs Type Indicator (MBTI). Katherine Briggs and Isabel Myers were a mother and daughter team who developed a tool on the back of some by Jung starting as early as 1923. Around the time of the Second World War, the personality assessment tool that they developed was used to guide the suitability of the women left behind for various types of roles. It has grown to become a building block in most leadership and management courses or in team building or as an exploratory tool to explore dysfunctional teams.

The licensing of the tool is tightly controlled and so I am unable to reprint it here but it is a worthwhile investment of your time and energy. There are four scales: extrovert–introvert; sensing–intuition; thinking–feeling, and judging–perceiving. The result of the assessment is a combination of four letters, for example, I'm an ENFJ.

In incredibly broad terms it examines where you get your energy from (others or on your own), whether you are a big picture or a detail person, whether you go with your heart or your head, and your preferred approach to prior planning. Before I start worrying about infringing copyright I shall stop there!

To describe myself I'd say I like to bounce ideas around with other people. I prefer to have an overview of what is going on, I need a vision of the whole. I tend to wear my heart on my sleeve and an empathic view of life is important to me. I like to be organized and I am often early.

Each trait is only a preference. It highlights areas you might need to work on and things that will come easily to you. It should not be held as an excuse for a particular behaviour. Looking at interactions between individuals, for example, you can learn how they might like information presented (written or verbal and big picture or fine detail).

The next tool to consider is Belbin.[21] This tool helps you identify your preferences for different team roles. Within a team it is helpful to have a range of preferences so that the full remit of options is covered. A team needs people who can generate new ideas and develop a vision, those that are happy to be team members and get the work done, those that like to help coordinate activities, some that like to drive things forward, and those that are good at detail and making sure things get finished. It is definitely worth investing time on the strengths and gaps of your team.

The final tool I think it is worth exploring is Honey and Mumford's preferred learning styles.[22] There are four broad categories plotted on two crossing axes. Your preferences are again, just that, only preferences and it doesn't mean that you can't learn in other ways, only how you prefer to learn. Whilst Donald Clark speaks rather derogatively about these tools, I am still a fan. The broad types can be considered by using a simple analogy but this is not substitute for the real thing. If I gave you a camera as a present, I would like you to think for a moment, what would you do first? Some of you might take it straight out of the box and start pressing the buttons (activist). Some of you might like to be shown by someone else how to use the camera and then you would happily get on with it (pragmatist). Some of you may start by reading the manual and only after that would you touch the camera (theorist). A final group might like to spend time thinking about the concept of photography (reflectors). My tongue is slightly in my cheek but I hope you are capturing a flavour of the concept.

Why do I think this is important? For me, there are two aspects both to do with developing self-awareness. If we are trying to create a 'learning' culture then surely to understand how best we learn may play a part. For a leader to understand the way their team likes to receive information and learn new things may be advantageous. It is also important if you are a teacher as you will find it easiest to teach within your preferred learning style. I challenge you to learn to teach in every style. I strongly believe that it is the trainer that should adjust to the preferred style of the learner. If you have a mixed group then you must put in something for everyone.

I would recommend that you do the full questionnaire and then spend some time thinking about how this might be relevant to your personal learning, your team role, your leading, and your teaching. It is not a gospel of how you must behave, simply use it as a tool to increase your self awareness and challenge yourself to grow your modus operandi.

OK, so you can start with your team homework. You now know your MBTI, Belbin, and Honey and Mumford preferences. So now what? Of course, there are a whole load of other tools you could use too! But I think that is enough to start things off. The next bit involves spending some time together and creating some 'ground rules' for the team. It works best if the team develop their own so that they have ownership of them and then you are more likely to get buy in. It lends itself well to the flipchart and sticky note method that has become the trademark of many an NHS training session! I loved the first three-quarters of Nancy Kline's book *Time to Think*.[23] She talks about developing a team who listen to each other and do not interrupt. She creates a system where everyone is given a turn to speak. Everyone must respectively listen to each of the ideas put forward. She also promotes a positive outlook on things which echoes my own value system. I am a strong believer in optimism, glass overflowing, high energy, praise, and appreciative enquiry. I think these techniques can lift a team, inspire it, and enthuse it to achieve.

Any more eye rolling when I mentioned ground rules? I'd love a better term for it if you have one.

What next?

We need to consider the roles of being a good 'follower' and what makes a good leader for our team.

Leadership

What is it?

There are so many books on leadership, each with its own model and definition. I am not going to go through all of them here but I will explore a handful of interesting ones.

There is now a leadership framework for the NHS which you can locate at <http://www.leadershipacademy.nhs.uk/lf>. It is due to be updated by the NHS Leadership Academy soon. There are a number of tools here for free including a 360-degree tool and a self-assessment tool.

The framework is divided into sections to look at:

- Setting direction

- Demonstrating personal qualities

- Working with others

- Managing services

- Improving services

- Creating the vision

- Delivering the strategy.

Within this chapter we are focusing on only some of those domains: demonstrating personal qualities and working with others. In my opinion, without those two, there is no team.

I would like you to consider this definition of leadership: 'the capacity to influence others'.

Leadership, using this definition, is nothing to do with position or hierarchy. So for those of you currently reading this thinking you are not a leader, I would say to you we all have the opportunity to influence others. I would like you to consider altering your self-perception ever so slightly to allow for the fact that you will be leading at times without even knowing.

There is no perfect leader. We should all be on a lifelong leadership journey.

I would like you to spend a couple of minutes considering a few famous leaders. Who do you find inspirational? Who might you aspire to be like? What are you basing your thoughts on? Which value system are you drawing on?

When I ask this question I often hear the names Ghandi and Mandela, but at some point we usually end up discussing Hitler. If I was to ask you how successful was Hitler in influencing others you would have to agree that he was incredibly effective at creating followers. It was his vision that was flawed (the master of the understatement!). So what was it that they have in common?

David Goleman[24] has done some interesting work. He describes the qualities of a good leader as:

- Self awareness

- Self-regulation

- Motivation

◆ Empathy

◆ Social skills.

This grouping sits well with my personal value system. If someone scored highly in each of those attributes then I would be happy to be led by them and I aspire to nurture these skills for when I am leading.

Goleman went further than this, he developed a series of styles of leadership for us to consider (see Figure 3.3).

It is said that a good leader can use four of these and does not just use one style. Two of the styles are considered to have a negative effect.

Guess what? The Hay Group has just published some work[25] that found the commonest style used by leaders across the NHS (both clinical and non-clinical alike!) was one of the detrimental styles! Only a very small proportion of our leaders could use the recommended four styles. There is work to be done!

As that is the commonest one and it's the one we are trying to avoid, let us start there. I need you to be really honest with yourself. If you recognize this style in yourself, that is the first step (self-awareness). The next step is mastering 'you' and trying to use an alternative style. This is the self-management phase (not so easy, but eminently doable with practice).

The Six Leadership Styles at a Glance

	Commanding	**Visionary**	**Affiliative**	**Democratic**	**Pacesetting**	**Coaching**
The leader's modus operandi	Demands immediate compliance	Mobilizes people toward a vision	Create harmony and builds emotional bonds	Forges consensus through participation	Sets high standards for performance	Develops people for the future
The style in a phrase	'Do what I tell you.'	'Come with me.'	'People come first.'	'What do you think?'	'Do as I do, now'	'Try this.'
Underlying emotional intelligence competencies	Drive to achieve, initiative, self-control	Self-confidence, empathy, change catalyst	Empathy, building relationships, communication	Collaboration, team leadership, communication	Conscientious-ness, drive to achieve, initiative	Developing others, empathy, self-awareness
When the style works best	In a crisis, to kick start a turnaround, or with problem employees	When changes require a new vision, or when a clear direction is needed	To heal rifts in a team or to motivate people during stressful circumstances	To build buy-in or consensus, or to get input from valuable employees	To get quick results form a highly motivated and competent team	To help an employee improve performance or develop long-term strengths
Overall impact on climate	Negative	Most strongly positive	Positive	Positive	Negative	Positive

Figure 3.3 Six leadership styles at a glance.
Reproduced with permission from Daniel Goleman, Leadership that Gets Results, *Harvard Business Review*, March–April 2000, pp. 82–83, Copyright © 2000 Harvard Business School Publishing. All rights reserved.

Whilst I am going to use the headings from Goleman, I'm going to build on each and put my own spin on them.

1. Pacesetting

I'm going to use a non-clinical example. I want you to imagine that my teenager is soon to go away to university and so I have decided that he needs to learn to cook an omelette. I am supervising him and I have already corrected him about the best way to crack the eggs. We are now at the whisking phase. I have taken over the whisking and the dialogue goes something like this, 'No, not like that. Let me show you. Tilt the bowl like this. Now watch the whisk action. See. Now . . . your turn!' By the time, I have taken over for the third time my son is now standing back from proceedings and his thumbs are getting their usual exercise on his mobile!

The effect of my behaviour has an impact on both of us. I am frustrated at his inability to complete such a simple task! He has learnt somewhere between nothing and very little. There is tension between us. He believes he can't do the task. He may not be willing to try and learn again. There is a negative atmosphere in the room that is palpable and will not aid future encounters.

Hmmm. Is it drafty? No? Never found yourself delegating something and then taking it back? Never secretly rolled your eyes or 'tutted' at someone else's standards or methods? 'They are just aren't up to your exacting high standards or working at your speed, so you'll do it yourself.' Fallen into the trap of micromanaging and unable to delegate? Be really honest with yourself.

I find it so easy to write about this style as I have witnessed so much of it!

From the results of the survey, it is highly probable that if you lead in the current NHS, that is highly likely to be your default style. We know it has a negative effect.

So what are you going to do to change it?

The next negative style is another one that all too common within certain areas of healthcare.

2. Commanding/coercive/directive

Whilst it is suggested by those people who are interested in leadership that this style is sometimes appropriate in a crisis, I would urge an element of caution with that approach.

This 'do it now', 'my way' with an instruction about how it is to be done but without a big picture view or context leaves the team absolutely laid open to a fixation error. We have already discussed the problem with this sort of steep hierarchy leadership. The followers are not empowered to challenge if they see the leader making a mistake. They are also not empowered to offer up their ideas, even though they may have years of useful experience.

The tasks within the type of crisis that we have already discussed are too complex to suit this style.

So, what should we be doing? All I've talked about so far is what not to do!

We need to grow our abilities in the next four styles. Try to identify which ones you already have in your 'Batman's utility belt' and see which ones you might need to develop.

3. Visionary/authoritative

In this style we can imagine some of the most famous leaders of the past. It is the ones who really master developing a clear, big picture and then take people with them that are the truly inspirational leaders.

This style is useful for long-term goals. There is a clear explanation of *why* this is the plan.

To develop this style you will need to work on your self-confidence and self-belief. There is a requirement to be able to show empathy and be a catalyst for change.[24]

4. Affiliative

This style puts the people before the task. It really builds the team. The emphasis is on harmony and working together and promoting good communication.[24]

For those of you who 'don't do fluffy bunny', there is clear evidence that if want to be a good leader, then you will have to learn. You will not have to function in this way all of time, but you should be able to use the style in the right setting. I commonly hear, 'I don't do feelings' and this is often accompanied by eye rolling. If you fail to master this skill, your team will suffer when there is conflict in the team and you are unable to either notice it or help to resolve it. The team will be less motivated and cope less well in times of stress or change as you may be oblivious to their needs. As we spend a large amount of the time in healthcare under high workload pressure and constantly moving political goal posts, we need the team to function under those conditions. We therefore need a leader who can support the team through these times. If you do master this style, the team will also feel valued and you never know, you might even generate a bit of loyalty in your team!

Still not convinced you might need to learn?

5. Democratic/collaborative

Often within healthcare there are lots of experts in a room that can all bring something to the table. This is just what this style encourages. It pools ideas from the whole team and encourages everyone to feel their ideas are valued. It works towards a consensus. By allowing everyone to contribute, it encourages commitment to the shared goal.

6. Coaching

This is where I confess that I'm a qualified coach and so I might have a slightly biased view of this approach!

I disagree with the words used in Figure 3.3 that are supposed to represent the coaching style. As a coach I would be highly unlikely to say, 'Try this' and much more likely to say, 'Would could you try next?' possibly followed by, 'What else?' The approach is designed to help the team to find their own solutions, not to tell them what to do.[24]

This style helps to improve performance and it is an investment in the long-term development of the team.[24]

Followership

There have been years of research into what makes an effective leader but that is only one team role. I think it is time to place more emphasis on the skills that are required for good followership. So what makes a good follower?

I am a strong believer in a positive mental attitude. On my team I like optimists. Whilst everyone can have an 'off' day and each of us will have difficult life events (e.g. bereavement, divorce, house move), there is no excuse for just being a negative person. You need to leave that attitude at the door and not bring it to work. Our patients in particular have every right to expect us to be positive with them. They should not know that we are tired or overworked. You may choose to share that with your closest team member but don't drag the whole team down with you.

I strongly believe our patients should never experience negativity from us in any form. As clichéd as it might sound, a smile costs you nothing and yet it can lift someone's mood if you make eye contact and give them a grin.

Why can't we just 'be in a good mood'? Since we are covering a few clichés, here is another one, 'Say no to no!'.

Say thank you! But do it in a genuine way that means something, not just a platitude. I will go through how to achieve this in depth later in the chapter.

On my team, I would like low-maintenance personalities. Here are a few ideas inspired by NASA when they are looking for a team.

Someone who:

◆ Puts groups goals ahead of personal goals

◆ Arrives on time

◆ Can both follow and lead

◆ Extroverted

◆ Optimistic

◆ Recognizes the needs of others

◆ Easily integrates

◆ Has good stress and anger management

◆ Is an effective listener

◆ Has a positive energy

◆ Communicates well

◆ Has can be creative

◆ Collaborates.

I don't think the creative bit has anything to do with sticky back plastic. I think it is more to do with new ideas and working within limited resources.

It is true to say that no matter how harmonious a team may be there will be times when conflict arises. Conflict, however, has a bad reputation. Conflict can be positive. Without a degree of challenge in a team and an expression of different ideas, progress will be far slower and it is possible to get stuck in a rut always moving in the same direction. Conflict can take many forms. It doesn't have to involve people raising their voices. Please remember though, that there is not a place for conflict in front of patients.

Conflict resolution

To illustrate the different ideas for resolving conflict, let's consider a non-clinical example. I want you to imagine that you are in the cinema. You have been waiting for weeks to see a new film and it has just been released. The cinema is fairly full but you had arrived early to get a good seat. You are settled in with your drink and your snack. The film starts. Unfortunately there are two people sitting in front of you who are having a loud conversation and they are munching popcorn noisily. It is interfering with your enjoyment of the long-awaited film.

What would you do?

Let's explore a few options. See if you can name each of the following approaches:

1. You either stand up or tap them on the shoulder and tell them in no uncertain terms to 'Be quiet!' or words to that effect but perhaps less polite. They raise their voices back at you and you end up in a full-blown argument. But they eventually back down when you mention your black belt in martial arts.

    Answer: Aggressive.
    This is an example of I win/you lose.

2. You 'tut' and roll your eyes and 'humf' but they don't hear you so you decide to put up with it. You might even consider kicking the back of the chair now and again.

    Answer: Accommodating (but with a bit of passive aggressive thrown in as we Brits have a tendency to do).
    This is an example of I lose/you win.

3. You get so exasperated that you decide to go and ask for a refund. The manager gives you the refund and in addition, decides to go and remove the people who are talking.

    Answer: Avoiding.
    This has resulted in a case of I lose/you lose.

4. You sheepishly tap them on the shoulder and negotiate that they will move a few places to the left and that you will move a few seats to the right. Neither of you will have such a good view. At least you will be able to hear the film and they can go and annoy someone else!

    Answer: Compromising.
    I both win and lose. You both win and lose.

5. You gently interrupt them. Using a calm tone of voice you begin by describing the behaviour. ('I have been waiting to see this film for weeks. When you are talking and eating popcorn, I am struggling to hear the film.') You then describe the impact their behaviour is having on you using an 'I' statement. ('I feel disappointed and a bit frustrated that I can't hear it.') Then ask them if they could do it differently. ('Do you think you could whisper instead?') They apologize as they hadn't realized they were bothering you and they offer you a piece of popcorn as a peace offering.

    We will return to this model later in the chapter, it is called SBIC.
    This stands for Situation Behaviour Impact Change (or Continue).
    Answer: Assertive.
    This results in a win/win. This is the solution that we are looking for.

People often refer to someone as being 'very assertive' when they actually mean aggressive. Assertive in the true sense of the word means expressing what you would like in a non-emotional way. Assertiveness is an essential skill to acquire. If you are in the role of being the patient's advocate or you can see an error about to happen, it is vital that you say something.

There are times to '**just speak up**' as just described and there are times to '**just be quiet**'. If someone has to perform a task that has a high cognitive workload, they may need peace and quiet in order to achieve this optimally. We can use the example of a surgeon who has to do a difficult bowel anastomosis or the paediatrician who has to work out complex drug doses for a 2.5 kg neonate where there is no room for even the tiniest of errors in either occasion. If the surgeon, or the paediatrician, runs an assertive briefing exercise prior to starting the task, they can explain, 'When I'm doing this bit of the task, I'll need everyone to be quiet so that I can concentrate'.

Standing up to someone where there is a perceived large power differential (steep hierarchy) requires self-confidence, self-belief, the right tools, and a bit of 'umph'. It is like any skill or muscle; it needs exercising and improves with practice.

Situation
Behaviour
'I' for Impact and 'I' for 'I' statement
Change (or Continue)

SBI is used by several organizations including the Centre for Creative Leadership, USA, The Performance Coach, UK and The Oxford School of Coaching and Mentoring (OCM). It is difficult to identify the original origin of the work and exactly how and by whom the modifications were made hence I include credits here to all three organizations.

If you think you might not be very assertive and you would find it difficult to challenge those people who are senior to you. The very first step is to think about how you feel in different settings and start rehearsing your 'I' statements:

◆ I felt uncomfortable

◆ I felt disappointed

◆ I felt frustrated

◆ I felt let down

◆ I felt saddened.

I don't want you to use my words though; I want you to find your own. It may be that you can think back to situations that have already happened. It may be, however, that you will have to have a 'dance floor and balcony' moment the next time you observe some less than ideal behaviour.

There are alternative versions of the conflict model that I've just introduced. There is one that uses a tank to represent the aggressive, a sniper (someone who undermines or who makes negative remarks, 'We've already tried that!' Skies eyes and sighs!) which represents the lose/lose, a doormat for the win/lose but the assertive is simply called win/win. There is also an analogy using different animals for each style (the owl, tortoise, and snake are used fairly regularly with a spattering of rhino and buffalo and donkey!).

Conflict does not have to involve people shouting at each other. As you can now see, it may be that people are just avoiding each other or the issue. Conflict can often build up over time and if it isn't resolved it can have an ongoing negative impact. The unresolved issues simply resurface later.

Remember that your use of language in a conflict setting can be important. For example, instead of saying, 'I disagree', try saying, 'We disagree'. I'll leave you to think about why those two options might have a different impact.

Coping with an angry outburst

If someone is having a full-on rant, assuming you are not in danger (in which case, I would remove yourself from the situation), then I would encourage you to listen. Listen carefully and actively. Eventually they will run out of steam. Use silence and just wait.

If you need to be uttering a secret mantra in your head then try something along the lines of:

'Maintain EQ. Listen. Deep breath. Maintain EQ and repeat . . .' (where EQ means emotional intelligence as explained earlier).

This is performed with an active listening type poker face. No smile but not a blank look either. Sit still, open your posture and don't fidget. Balance the amount of eye contact you use. The eye contact should be enough to show that you are listening but not too intense that it becomes a staring competition.

I absolutely do not agree that you should match their volume. I think that by speaking quietly, it brings down the energy in the room and they have to listen harder if they are going to hear what you have to say. The real red rag to a bull phrase is to tell someone to calm down. You will find it is more like pouring petrol on the flames!

Acknowledge the emotion. 'You seem upset, shall we find somewhere more private to talk about it?' or if you are already somewhere suitable replace that bit with, 'would you like to talk about it?'.

It is worth summarizing what you have heard. There are a few techniques for accomplishing this. It is worth stating which of these you are using—this is called 'pre-framing'. For example, 'So, what I've heard so far is/I think you said/ Using my words, what I've heard so far is/To summarize . . . ' So you can either use the other person's words which you have remembered verbatim (reflecting). Or you can use your own words (paraphrasing). Or you can pull all of the ideas together into a list as a summary (not surprisingly known as summarizing).

And then you need to check that you have got it right. Clarify that you have it correct by asking a few questions to see how accurate your listening has been. Also look for non-verbal communication to see how what you said has been received. You need to establish if there is some more information: 'Was there something else involved?', 'What else may have contributed?', 'Are we missing anything?'.

The next step is to ask them what would help rather than to just try and jump in to fix it. We often take a very paternalistic view of things in healthcare. It is not meant in a negative way, we want to help people (for a large number of us that was why we went into healthcare). Avoid this desire to 'rescue'. This can be achieved by asking them: 'What do you think might help?', 'What are the possible solutions?', 'What would you like to see happen next?', 'Where should we go from here?'. They will know what they need better than we do, you just need to help them explore their own solutions.

If they get stuck, try summarizing the story so far as a way of almost playing it back to them. It can sometimes help to hear it spoken by someone else.

Only after they have decided what they need should we offer up ourselves as part of the solution. 'Is there something you would like me to do?'

At this point summarize again but this time listing solutions and not problems. You then need to close the conversation. Check you have agreement with the actions. Agree whether you are going to have a further meeting and a timescale for that if appropriate. If you will not be involved again establish who will be involved in the follow-up. A really clear plan with consensus can save a lot of trouble later. Consider documenting it if that fits the situation. This is best completed while you are both still there and sign it to say that you both agreed to it. This, of course, is too formal for many instances so you will have to use your judgement.

Prevention is better than cure

In addition to the obvious personality interactions, a few other sources of conflict which were reported in our study are listed here. This part of the list looks at problems with team behaviours:

- Unclear team roles
- Preferred team role taken by another
- Perceived unfairness
- Perceived versus actual power
- Accountability (lack of or lack of clarity of)
- Approach to change
- Difference in preferred communication styles
- Difference in preferred learning styles
- Mixed messages
- Preconceived ideas and conflicting expectations.

If you are leading a team it may be worth you spending time considering these in the context of your team.

This list is the result of complex team dynamics. The next step is to break behaviour down a bit more. Next is a list taken from the SHEEP sheet of all of the types of individual behaviours that our participants felt had a negative impact on them and hence may be a source of conflict:

- Challenging (negative) behaviour
- Lack of diversity consideration (gender, sex, culture)
- Prejudice
- Aggression
- Laziness
- Rudeness
- Snobbery
- Dishonesty
- Lack of consideration
- Lack of respect
  - of others
  - by others
- Over familiarity
- Empire building

- Trying to impress

- Negative responses

- Loss of sense of humour

- Unwillingness

- Apathy

- Fear

- Insecurity

- Making assumptions

- Reluctance to change

- Malicious intent.

Let's explore some of those in more detail. We have already alluded to the downward spiral that can follow negativity. For me, we can group into that loss of sense of humour and unwillingness.

There is no place at work, in my view, for apathy and laziness. These definitely represent a 'button' for me. If you are being paid to perform a task then I think you should perform it to the best of your ability. If the task is boring or not engaging enough, then either it should be broken up into smaller chunks or shared amongst different people. It can perhaps be interspersed with something more exciting but . . . I feel like I'm entering mummy mode . . . 'I'm afraid it still has to be done and moaning about it won't make it go away'. I am not suggesting you enter mummy mode with your team, in fact, quite the contrary; we should avoid switching into parent–child mode. I would recommend coaching mode instead. Perhaps something more along the lines of, 'How could you do it differently?' or 'What would make it more exciting/more manageable?'.

If the laziness is not task related but generally a whole attitude to the job, then don't avoid it. Name the behaviour and talk about the impact that it is having on you and on team moral using the SBIC model above. Nip it in the bud early. If it continues to be a problem then you need to tackle it as it will have a damaging effect on the whole team if you are seen to condone it.

There are two absolutes on the list: malicious intent and dishonesty do not belong in the health service. We also need to remove prejudice and discrimination.

Respect?

What does that mean for you?

Let's start with staff. How will you know when another member of staff is respecting you or your wishes? How can you show the people you work with that you respect them?

What to do when you are on the receiving side of poor behaviour

Do you know what type of behaviour pushes your buttons? How will you identify when something is winding you up? Where do you feel it first? Then what happens?

The earlier you can identify it, the earlier you can take control of it and put in some self-management. What are you going to do to try and intervene? Are you going to be assertive and explain the impact that the behaviour is having on you? Are you going to walk away and avoid it? Will you try the 'two-breath technique' where for 5 seconds you say nothing and you simply take two deep breaths and let all the negativity disperse. How will you choose which option to adopt in each setting?

Whilst walking away is preferable to raised voices, I would like you to consider adopting the SBIC model that was mentioned earlier.

Situation
Behaviour
'I' for Impact and 'I' for 'I' statement
Change (or Continue).

The first step is to think about where you are going to have the conversation, remembering as earlier highlighted, that curtains are not soundproof and that the conversation should not take place in front of patients. Choose a suitable private venue or situation.

The next letter encourages you to focus on the behaviour. Remember that personality is fairly set once you pass your early twenties but personality is not an excuse for poor behaviour. In the iceberg analogy, the part of the iceberg that is under the water represents personality, and the part that is visible above the water line is the behaviour. Everyone can follow minimum standards of acceptable behaviour. It is the behaviour and only the behaviour that you are going to comment on.

You need to give a short description of what you observed. (This is not a tool for hearsay.) Keep it factual and not emotional. Do not accuse the other person of something and choose your words carefully. Watch your body language. You are not sitting in judgement.

I want you to pay close attention to how you felt when you observed the behaviour. This is very important to make the next bit work. This is the 'I' statement that we introduced earlier. It describes the impact that the behaviour had on you when you observed it. Do not fall into the trap of second guessing how other people felt. This can be disputed and gives the person behaving poorly an option to argue with you. We are not trying to start an argument.

'I felt uncomfortable' is a good example but you must use the words that describe how you actually felt at the time.

The next bit involves asking them, 'How might you have done it differently?'. The idea here is that to change behaviour you are more likely to be successful if you can encourage the person to 'own' the change. It may be that you cannot get them to come up with the change in which case I would then tell them the alternative behaviour and then explore it with them.

The observant amongst you will have noticed that it said Change or Continue. This model can be used to praise. In this setting you wish to reinforce the positive behaviour and encourage it to continue.

I usually encourage people to begin using the model with praise. Once you have mastered the model, I suggest you try your first few times using it to tackle poor behaviour with your peer group. Once you are confident with the model, then is the time to work on more ingrained behaviour.

I think it is best to consider an example at this stage. Let's imagine that there is a ward round. The ward round is being led by the Registrar equivalent and there is a Senior Sister, a Foundation level (F1) (house officer equivalent), and an F2 (or senior house officer equivalent) also present. You are also attending the ward round. The Registrar is rather cutting to the F1 when they present the history of the first patient. After the second presentation, there is some 'tutting' and 'skying' of eyes from the Registrar. No one else has said anything and they are all behaving like this is a normal everyday occurrence.

Have you intervened yet? If not, why not? For those of you who have not yet stepped in, is it because you witness behaviour like that or worse regularly? Is it because you feel it is not your place? Is it because you wouldn't know what to say?

For any of you, that still don't feel you should step in:

> Do you think this is how we should teach our junior doctors?
> Is it an example of a learning culture?
> What did the patients think?

I think the intervention should resemble something like this, but you should use your own words not mine.

Situation

Where should we have the conversation? Take a moment to plan it. How about when we have finished in this bay?

> Spoken very quietly to the Registrar, 'Can we talk out of earshot for a minute?'. If they try to decline, 'It will be very quick, but it's important'. Move to an office if available, but at the very least to a private space.

Behaviour and impact with 'I' statement

Have a think what you might say. If you have time, write it down.

> I would go for something along the lines of, 'When you spoke to . . . insert name of F1, not just their title . . . in that way, I was a bit taken aback'.

Change

What are going to say next?

> My line would be, 'How could you have done it differently?'. If that was met with blank looks or the floor suddenly becoming very interesting, then I would add, 'What is important when creating a good learning environment for . . . person's name?'.

This whole conversation could potentially happen in under 2 minutes.

1. 'When you spoke to . . . insert name of F1, not just their title . . . in that way, I was a bit taken aback.'

2. 'How could you have done it differently?'

With the time pressure that we under, it is a common excuse used to let poor behaviour slide. Another common excuse is that 'so and so' is always like. Well, not anymore. We need to stop this behaviour.

It is bad enough to staff, but to our patients in it unforgivable!

Our care should begin with a smile from the time when they first arrive on the ward/reception/clinic. Not the feeling that you are too busy, when no one looks up from what they are doing. We need to make each patient know they are important to us. We need to imagine each one is to be treated like our friend or family member.

Whilst I realize that the 'family and friends' test is currently being used as a political angle, the 'grandmother test' was taught to me as a medical student over 20 years ago. (*My children are convinced that I pre-date cars and television. I don't, but I suspect the 'grandmother test' might be that old.*)

Praise

> *There is no such whetstone, to sharpen a good wit and encourage a will to learning, as is praise*

Roger Ascham (1515–1568), *The Schoolmaster* (1570) book 1

We do not praise people often enough. There is good evidence that praise can raise moral and that better moral can improve efficiency (see work from Professor Michael West's group). I have already alluded to the fact that it needs to be specific and that tailor made to be of real value. As I've suggested earlier, we can use the **SBIC** model to deliver it.

Why do we need to move away from non-specific platitudes? Does it really matter how it is delivered as long as we say 'well done'? Yes!

There is an unfortunately rather common way of giving feedback within large sections of the NHS. It is known as a sandwich, the filling of which I'm far too polite to mention here. It is suggested that you wish to give someone some very negative feedback so in order to make it more palatable, it is served up with a layer of bread on each side to hide the taste! The bread takes the form of false praise or platitudes. It would usually start something along the lines of, 'You are doing a great job' or 'You did that really well'. Then there is a pause and an intake of breath, 'BUT . . . ' and then the criticism is delivered in a dollop. It has been a Pavlovian conditioning response that after praise (which they now ignore), they just wait for the criticism.

After the criticism, another piece of bread is served to try and cover up the bit in the middle.

Patients

What about our patients? We have alluded to the fact that they should be central to everything we do. Every decision we make should bear them in mind, no matter how far removed you might feel from them. Some of you will have direct contact with patients; others of you will have a role that seems more removed. Whatever your role, I want you to maintain sight of our real purpose in the health service, the quality care, safety, and experience of the patient.

If we consider the patient to be a central component of every team (yes, clichéd, but no apologies), then let's review the SHEEP sheet list again, but think about it with our patients in mind: Challenging (negative) behaviour, Lack of diversity consideration (gender, sex, culture), Prejudice, Aggression, Laziness, Rudeness, Snobbery, Dishonesty, Lack of consideration, Lack of respect of others and by others, Overfamiliarity, Empire building, Trying to impress, Negative responses, Loss of sense of humour, Unwillingness, Apathy, Fear, Insecurity, Making assumptions, Reluctance to change, and Malicious intent.

How do these behaviours that we have heard are happening in healthcare, compare to how the GMC[26] suggests we should behave? Listed here are the GMC guidelines for good practice:[26]

◆ Make the care of your patient your first concern.

◆ Provide a good standard of practice and care.

  ○ Keep your professional knowledge and skills up to date.

  ○ Recognize and work within the limits of your competence.

◆ Take prompt action if you think that patient safety, dignity, or comfort is being compromised.

◆ Protect and promote the health of patients and the public.

◆ Treat patients as individuals and respect their dignity.

  ○ Treat patients politely and considerately.

  ○ Respect patients' right to confidentiality.

◆ Work in partnership with patients.

  ○ Listen to, and respond to, their concerns and preferences.

  ○ Give patients the information they want or need in a way they can understand.

  ○ Respect patients' right to reach decisions with you about their treatment and care.

  ○ Support patients in caring for themselves to improve and maintain their health.

◆ Work with colleagues in the ways that best serve patients' interests.

◆ Be honest and open and act with integrity.

◆ Never discriminate unfairly against patients or colleagues.

◆ Never abuse your patients' trust in you or the public's trust in the profession.

  Reproduced with permission from the General Medical Council.

Let's consider a few of the contrasts between how we should be behaving and what we have heard happens in reality.

Respect

How can we show our patients respect?

My answer would begin by getting the basics right. We need to think about their basic physiological needs—to be 'fed and watered', to be clean themselves and in a clean environment that is at the right temperature.

We need to do everything we can to preserve their dignity and privacy.

We can smile and be in a positive frame of mind. We can care and keep our patients safe. We can find out how our patient would like to be addressed and personalize their care.

We need to listen. We need to ask the right questions and then we need to listen some more. There is no place for rudeness, prejudice, or discrimination. We need to show some empathy.

Example 3.1 Out of the mouths of babes

Later today I am due to take my 4-year-old daughter to see the GP. At breakfast this morning she had some questions for me about it. I was shocked at their content.

'Mummy, will anyone be able to hear what I am saying when I see the doctor?'

'No, we will be in a room on our own, just you and mummy and the doctor', I reply.

'Will she be able to tell anyone what I've told her?' she added.

'Actually it's a man doctor, is that ok?' and I wait and watch her.

She paused for a moment, 'Yes'.

I add, 'And doctors are not allowed to tell anyone what patients tell us, we have to keep it a secret!'. A huge smile and look of relief wash over her. She considers her health issue to be very private and did not want to share it with 'just anyone'.

I sat there and studied her for a while, wondering how on earth she had become so insightful at the ripe old age of 4! Why is it that we, as healthcare professionals, still rely on 'magic curtains' to suddenly soundproof a bed? Why, when the basic ideas of **confidentiality** and **respect** are obviously childlike, are we still getting it wrong?

For those of you who are not naturally empathic, have a real go at asking yourself, 'What would I want for myself or my partner or my child or my grandmother?' I would like to share with you something from my family (see Example 3.1).

Shared decision-making

The decision making that we have explored in this chapter should involve our patients when possible (I realize this is not possible in an emergency when they are semiconscious). This involves presenting information in a way that they can understand it. Giving them time to process the information and ask questions. It would also include helping them to review the decisions that have been made as new information becomes available. DODAR still applies; Diagnosis, Option generation, Decide, Assessment, and Review. This may also apply to working alongside patients' relatives.

Shared understanding

We need to make sure that we have a shared mental model with our patients. When information is being transferred in either direction (patient to healthcare professional or vice versa) we need to double check that this transfer has been successful.

There is another important aspect of information flow that helps us to have shared expectations. Within healthcare, we will always have limited resources. Not every patient can be first on an operating list. We will never have enough nurses for every patient to have individual care all day long. Not every patient can be the first in the GP surgery that day or the first to be seen in the outpatient clinic. This invariably means that there will be some waiting. Whilst I am a big fan of streamlining processes and improving efficiency we will always be constrained by resources. I think this is when it is vital that we are honest with our patients.

However, by honesty, I do not mean become a 'mood hoover'. I do not mean that we should burden our patients with facts like we are overworked or understaffed. See Examples 3.2, 3.3 and 3.4.

Example 3.2 Honesty and expectation

An honest letter before the clinic that states how long you can expect to be at the hospital and explains the systems, allows our patients to plan their lives, by explaining it will be necessary to see a doctor who may want some tests taken and an x-ray performed. These tests are performed in different parts of the hospital so it will be necessary to move to those different departments before returning back to the main clinic.

Example 3.3 More honesty and expectations

By explaining that on the emergency surgery list, sometimes there is a patient with a life-threatening emergency that queue jumps and may mean they will have to wait a bit longer, we are creating a shared mental model with our patient.

Example 3.4 Expectation and shared mental model

By saying it should happen in the late morning but it might be lunchtime by the time you get your scan rather than the scan is booked at 11.15 am; again we are being honest and hopefully trying to create a shared understanding of the constraints that we work with.

Team working and leadership

By envisaging that our patient and perhaps their relatives, are part of the team with whom we are we working, perhaps we can start to realize a new model of care. A truly patient-centric approach would allow both the patients and relatives input into the decision-making. This model would involve a less paternalistic view of doctor–patient interaction where 'doctor knows best'. Again the approachability of the staff and perceived power-distance (hierarchy) would come into play.

How will you ensure that all your colleagues work well with the patient too? See Example 3.5.

Example 3.5 Staff expectations of a patient

It is handover. You are told that the patient in bed 2 is Mrs Smith. You are told that she is very demanding and her daughter is difficult.

How do you feel now? Are you able to wipe the slate clean and offer the best possible care for Mrs Smith? How are you expecting a meeting with her daughter to be? How might that affect the interaction?

What can you do to help unpick and then diffuse this situation?

Try asking questions and then listening. Are they scared? Have they had all the information they need? Are we missing something? Is there a problem with our care? How could we make it better? What would help?

How can you make sure you do not alter the expectations or care of one of your patients when you are 'handing them over'?

These cycles of negativity can be self-perpetuating. I encourage you to break them. Remain the optimist and lift the room, however challenging that may be. I believe the negative labels that are sometimes given to patients or their relatives can actually affect the standard of their care and even increase the chance of an error occurring.

Situational awareness

How will you make it 'safe' for your patient to challenge your decisions? How will you encourage your patient to be part of the processes that could tailor-make their care? How will you check you are getting it right? How will you encourage them to review decisions as new information becomes available? How will you help them plan and anticipate their next steps?

How will you maintain your knowledge and skills to make sure the care for this patient is as good as it can be? How will you know if you need to ask for help and where the limits of your competence may lie?

Time to think

So, assuming you are not perfect, what could you improve upon?

What negative impact might you inadvertently be having on your team and what are you going to do about it? What will that change look like? How will you know when you achieved it?

How are you going to bring in more praise and make it meaningful? Can you draw on examples of when it has worked before?

A few questions to help you mull things over

1. What is the ideal hierarchy gradient between the leader and the followers within a team?

    A. Flat (All the same, 0°)

    B. 90°

C. 45°

D. 15°

E. Debbie I haven't got a clue what you're talking about!

ANSWER

D 15°

If you're leading a team it's a good idea to make sure you're approachable. This means if you're about to make a mistake your team will feel able to challenge you.

However, whilst collaboration is great, a completely flat hierarchy is not ideal either as no one is responsible for making the final decision.

2. The best approach(es) to conflict resolution involves:

A. Avoidance

B. Aggression

C. Assertiveness

D. Accommodating

E. Compromise

ANSWER

'C' is the best answer, aiming for the win/win. This is not always possible and it may be necessary to look at 'E' compromising. There are times when you do not feel strongly about something, that it is better on that occasion to be accommodating 'D' and back down on this more minor point, to invest in a long-term goal. If you feel the situation is too emotional for either party, then avoidance 'A' until everything has settled down may be preferable. The answer that is never acceptable is aggression. If it does occur towards you, think about your personal safety first, but if that is not at risk, maintain your own emotional intelligence and do not get sucked in to being agressive yourself.

3. You arrive at an emergency and it is a bit chaotic. No one seems to have clear roles and no one seems to be coordinating things. What would you do?

A. Work out who should be in charge and tell them to lead it

B. Take charge yourself

C. Give them some time and hope that a leader will emerge

D. Tell them you are calling their boss

E. Ask, 'Who is leading?'

I think that E may be a good place to start. Other options may be necessary depending on who is present and what the situation is, but by asking the question it might get people to start thinking about leadership.

With enough people present, it should be possible to also ask about everyone's roles. Is someone keeping time, for example? 'What would you like me to do?' might be a good question. Other questions to have up your sleeve include:

'Which algorithm/guideline are we using here?'
'How long have the . . . e.g. *saturations been low*?'
'What is the diagnosis here?'
'What are we missing?'
'What else could it be?'
'Do we have all the right people/equipment that we need?'
'What are the next steps?'
'Can we review where we are?'

Key points from Chapters 1–3

◆ We all make mistakes. Are you looking at how to avoid your next one?

◆ We need to embed an open culture. Culture is one of many informal systems in which we function.

◆ There should be an inquisitive approach to error that seeks out the learning and shares it: the learning culture.

◆ This should include 'memory checks' and 'safety events'.

◆ The new error checklist—the SHEEP sheet—helps gather more information following an actual event or a nearly event. It is quick and easy to use.

◆ The SHEEP sheet can be used for trend analysis.

◆ Information flow across an organization can be achieved using a brief/debrief model using Debbie's Diamond.

◆ Systems errors are commonly part of the holes in the Swiss cheese and should feature in the solutions for improved safety.

◆ Things are not always what they seem: avoid assumption.

◆ 'What am I missing here?' is a healthy question to keep asking.

◆ If the hierarchy is too steep, the team will not feel able to challenge the leader when they are making a mistake. We all make mistakes.

- If there is a flat hierarchy, no natural leader emerges, ask the question, 'Who's leading?'

- Followership is a much overlooked and important skill to have. This can involve being assertive enough to speak up if things are about to go wrong.

- We will all push someone else's buttons. We can't change the other person, only ourselves.

- We need to become more aware of how we are impacting on others (increase our self-awareness). This might begin with knowing our preferred learning style, team role and our personality type (MBTI).

- Once we know who we are more likely to 'clash' with, we can try and blend in a bit better (self-management) to avoid conflict.

- If we do end up in conflict we will behave in an assertive way (this is completely different from aggressive although the terms are often misused) and aim to find a win–win situation.

- A good leader will be able to switch to using four different leaderships styles when appropriate and will avoid micro-management or pacesetting. This pacesetting style currently dominates the NHS in both clinical and non-clinical leaders.

- Remember when giving feedback and praise:

  - Situation Behaviour Impact Change or Continue.

References

1. Buttigieg SC, West MA, Dawson JF. Well-structured teams and the buffering of hospital employees from stress. *Health Services Management Research* 2011;24(4):203–12.
2. Gaba DM. Crisis resource management and teamwork training in anaesthesia. *British Journal of Anaesthesia* 2010;105(1):3–6.
3. Holzman RS, Cooper JB, Gaba DM, Philip JH, Small SD, Feinstein D. Anesthesia crisis resource management: real-life simulation training in operating room crises. *Journal of Clinical Anesthesia* 1995;7(8):675–87.
4. Howard SK, Gaba DM, Fish KJ, Yang G, Sarnquist FH. Anesthesia crisis resource management training: teaching anesthesiologists to handle critical incidents. *Aviation, Space, and Environmental Medicine* 1992;63(9):763–70.
5. Reznek M, Smith-Coggins R, Howard S, Kiran K, Harter P, Sowb Y, *et al*. Emergency medicine crisis resource management (EMCRM): pilot study of a simulation-based crisis management course for emergency medicine. *Academic Emergency Medicine* 2003;10(4):386–9.

6. Reader T, Flin R, Lauche K, Cuthbertson BH. Non-technical skills in the intensive care unit. *British Journal of Anaesthesia* 2006;96(5):551–9.

7. David M. Gaba SKH, Kevin J. Fish, Brian E. Smith, Yasser A. Sowb. *Simulation & Gaming* June 2001;32(2):175–93.

8. van Avermaete JAG, Kruijsen E. *The evaluation of non-technical skills of multi-pilot aircrew in relation to the JAR-FCL requirements* (Project rep.: CR-98443). Amsterdam, The Netherlands; 1998.

9. Flin RH, Martin L, Goeters K-M, Hormann J, Amalberti R, Valot C, *et al.* Development of the NOTECHS (Non-Technical Skills) system for assessing pilots' CRM skills. *Journal of Human Performance in Extreme Environments* 2003;3:95–117.

10. Mitchell L, Flin R, Yule S, Mitchell J, Coutts K, Youngson G. Evaluation of the Scrub Practitioners' List of Intraoperative Non-Technical Skills system. *International Journal of Nursing Studies* 2012;49(2):201–11.

11. Johnston PW, Fioratou E, Flin R. Non-technical skills in histopathology: definition and discussion. *Histopathology* 2011;59(3):359–67.

12. Bahl R, Murphy DJ, Strachan B. Non-technical skills for obstetricians conducting forceps and vacuum deliveries: qualitative analysis by interviews and video recordings. *European Journal of Obstetrics, Gynecology, and Reproductive Biology* 2010;150(2):147–51.

13. Flin R, Patey R. Non-technical skills for anaesthetists: developing and applying ANTS. *Best Practice & Research. Clinical Anaesthesiology* 2011;25(2):215–27.

14. Flin R, Patey R, Glavin R, Maran N. Anaesthetists non-technical skills. *British Journal of Anaesthesia* 2010;105(1):38–44.

15. Yule S, Flin R, Maran N, Rowley D, Youngson G, Paterson-Brown S. Surgeons non-technical skills in the operating room: reliability testing of the NOTSS behavior rating system. *World Journal of Surgery* 2008;32(4):548–56.

16. Fletcher G, Flin R, McGeorge P, Glavin R, Maran N, Patey R. Anaesthetists Non-Technical Skills (ANTS): evaluation of a behavioural marker system. *British Journal of Anaesthesia* 2003;90(5):580–8.

17. DONCS assessments. <https://training.rcpsych.ac.uk/information-about-doncs-assessments>.

18. Kelly CA, Upex A, Bateman DN. Comparison of consciousness level assessment in the poisoned patient using the alert/verbal/painful/unresponsive scale and the Glasgow Coma Scale. *Annals of Emergency Medicine* 2004;44(2):108–13.

19. Teasdale G, Jennett B. Assessment of coma and impaired consciousness. A practical scale. *Lancet* 1974;2(7872):81–4.

20. Bromiley Report verdict and corrected timeline. <http://www.chfg.org/resources/07_qrt04/Anonymous_Report_Verdict_and_Corrected_Timeline_Oct_07.pdf>.

21. Belbin M. *Management Teams*. London: Heinemann; 2001.

22. Honey P, Mumford A. *The Learning Styles Questionnaire, 80-item version*. Maidenhead, UK: Peter Honey Publications; 2006.

23. Kline N. *Time to Think: Listening to Ignite the Human Mind*. New York: Cassell Illustrated; 1998.

24. Goleman D. What makes a leader? *Harvard Business Review* 1998;76(6):93–102.

25. Hay Group website: <http://www.haygroup.com>.

26. GMC. *Duties of a doctor*. <http://www.gmc-uk.org/guidance/good_medical_practice/duties_of_a_doctor.asp>.

4

The 'E' of SHEEP: Environment

The art of being wise is the art of knowing what to overlook

William James (1842–1910)

The Principles of Psychology (1890), Volume 2, Chapter 22

Let's start by exploring the first 'E' of the algorithm (see Figure 4.1).

Dynamic versus Static

Patients—dynamic

If we consider our patients, some of them will be admitted to a ward and they may spend their time entirely on that ward. Others may require 'journeys' for investigations such as x-rays and scans or something more invasive like endoscopy or surgery.

If they are admitted as an emergency trauma case they may arrive via ambulance and spend time in the Emergency Department with a journey to CT scan and then on to theatre and after theatre either to recovery or ICU (Intensive Care Unit), prior to returning to a ward.

An outpatient visit may involve a 'journey' from outpatients to have an x-ray or ultrasound scan or an ECG (electrocardiogram or heart tracing) and blood tests and then back to outpatients.

We need to consider how efficient and safe these 'journeys' can be. It makes sense at a design phase when building a hospital to think about the proximity of areas such as the Emergency Department, the CT scanner, theatre, and ICU. However, once the hospital is built there is not a huge amount we can do to alter the efficiency of the distances we must cover in this setting. For anyone who has, like me, struggled to push a sick patient in a bed with a portable ventilator, a portable monitor, and a series of pumps along a corridor, the actual size of the

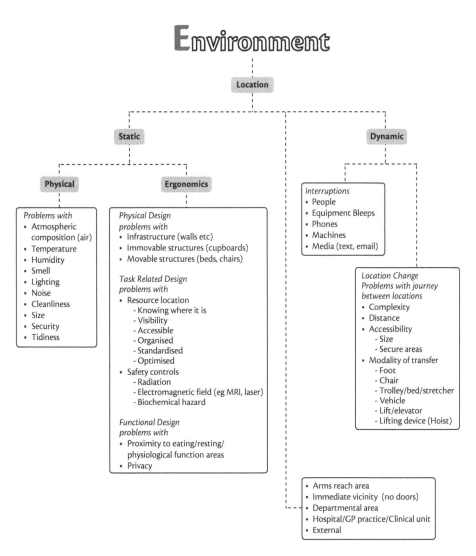

Figure 4.1 'E'—the SHEEP model.

corridors and the doors is of great relevance. But again, once it is designed, it is difficult to alter. However, it is hampered further if the corridor seems to have been converted into a storage area for spare beds and trolleys. Then there is the joy of taking that fully laden bed into a lift, which again is not normally big enough. A further soapbox moment can be found in Box 4.1.

For those of you who cannot relate to what I'm currently describing I would like you to imagine that you are coming with me.

> # Box 4.1 Soapbox moment
>
> My first plea is to those of you who may be involved in hospital design. Please, in the future can we think more fully about which departments should be close together from a patient safety perspective (not staff convenience)? Please can we make the corridors and doors and lifts big enough?
>
> My second plea is that we don't use the corridors as a storage area, so again when we design the hospital, if we need a bed and trolley store can we factor that in please?

The very sick patient that we are transferring from the ward needs to go to ICU urgently. The patient is already intubated (tube into their windpipe) and ventilated (on a breathing machine). The breathing machine sticks out from the end of the bed and we need a large oxygen cylinder to give oxygen to the patient and to make the ventilator work. We always take a backup of a self-inflating bag (Ambu or equivalent) in case the ventilator fails and we need to breathe for the patient by hand instead. We have a portable monitor on the end of the bed facing us so that we can see all of their vital signs while we are moving along (things like blood pressure, heart rate, etc.). The screen of this is about the size of a small laptop. In addition, we might have drugs and drips, some of which might be in a pump (a device which moves the syringe at a rate which you can change, but the drug is being given continuously). These pumps are about the same length as a laptop but not as wide. If the patient is really sick we may also need a portable defibrillator (a machine that can deliver a shock to restart the heart) and a big bag of other equipment and drugs that we might use along the way.

In the middle of this melee is the patient (unconscious and very sick). They will have lots of tubes and drips—none of which you want to dislodge while you are moving along.

We need a porter (or ideally two) plus two appropriately trained clinical staff as a minimum. We are now in the lift. The patient's blood pressure is dropping and we need to give more of one of the drugs that are going through the pump. The staff member that is sandwiched down the side of the bed is just about close enough to the myriad of pumps that are attached to the patient.

How easy is it to identify which drug is in which pump in this setting? How easy is it to see the monitor from the angle you are standing at and yet it is vital if we are changing the dose of that medicine, that we watch the blood pressure on a beat-to-beat basis to titrate it to effect? How easy will it be to manage if one of the tubes comes loose? What if the lift fails? Will you have enough oxygen?

We need to plan our patient journeys thoroughly. We need to plan and antici-pate all of those possible problems and try to pre-empt them. We need to realize that moving a patient is an at-risk time. There should be a briefing of the plan before you leave the safe area and a debrief once you arrive in the next safe area to look for learning points.

From a patient perspective the signposting around the hospital should be clear enough. There should be regular maps displayed along the corridor. There should be adequate information sent out to our patients about where they are going in advance with maps. Details such as where to park or where public transport might arrive will ease the stress levels of our patients before their appointments. Adequately staffed welcome desks to direct people are essential. There should be adequate numbers and different forms of transport for within the hospital (wheelchairs and motorized vehicles). The wheelchairs need to be stored in a suitable area near each entrance. There needs to be a system that regularly restocks this store.

Colour coding of lines or signs or footprints on floors for regular journeys may be beneficial. It is far easier to explain to someone to follow the purple footprints. Hopefully we will soon employ technology to help us with internal tracking systems and perhaps internal 'sat nav' (satellite navigation) so that our patients don't get lost.

For now, wouldn't it be lovely if we knew that if any of our staff saw that some-one looked lost, they would stop what they were doing (yes, even if they were busy!) and take a moment to help them.

Patient journeys can also occur between NHS institutions. The directions again can be vitally important as well as knowing which part of the receiving institu-tion is the bit that you need (see Example 4.1). There can also be a problem accessing a secure area when you arrive in either a new department or new insti-tution. Perhaps there is a swipe card entry or a code and you find yourself stuck outside it with a sick patient!

Example 4.1 Knowing your environment

I was fairly new to transferring intensive care patients from one ICU to another. This involves taking a patient (similar to the one described earlier in the lift) in an ambulance from one town or city to another. The space in the back of an ambulance is not that large. For the transfer to be successful there is a huge amount of planning of equipment, oxygen supplies, monitor-ing equipment and battery supplies, drugs, notes, copies of x-rays, as well as the right staff for the job in case the patient deteriorates en route. I was proud of my organizational ability on this occasion. Everything had been checked by me and double checked by the staff member who was coming with me. The journey had been uneventful until we couldn't find the other hospital. When we finally found the other hospital we had three false starts at trying to leave the ambulance at three different entrances to the hospital and then spent ages wandering the corridors of an unknown hospital looking for the ICU! I am very much hoping that there can be learning from my mistakes.

Fortunately, apart from some early acquisition of grey hair as we wondered if the battery life on the monitor would be adequate and whether our oxygen calculations had a bit of extra built in, we survived intact.

It is a good idea to have a map (even if you have satellite navigation which did not exist when I was junior!). It is important to talk to the local team and ask which entrance you should come to and then how to get to the Unit. It is important to have the name of the person you are dealing with on that unit and a contact number. It is useful to phone them shortly before you arrive and to even ask if they could come down and meet you.

Do you have systems and checklists in place to help this process be reliable and repeatable? Is it systematic and easy to find a guideline and a checklist for transfers? Is having a map and entrance and contact and swipe access on the checklist? Who goes? How senior are they? Has everyone been trained? How often are they doing transfers? Are you reviewing any errors? Could you make it even safer? Where is it discussed? What about when the staff rotate?

Staff—dynamic

Whilst some staff may work just in one clinical area (single ward, clinic, theatre), others may cover vast areas (multiple wards, theatre and ICU, whole hospitals, or even multiple hospitals). Whilst some staff may have responsibility for large areas, this may be a more hands-off role whilst others literally spend their days traipsing along corridors.

It can be difficult to plan the day as the clinical priorities of varying patients at different stages of their care are never predictable. It is an interesting cognitive balance of planning tasks (list making and prioritizing) interspersed with the skill of being flexible enough to cope with changing workload and priorities over which there is no control (see Example 4.2).

Example 4.2 Junior doctor

Imagine in this example that you have the role of the junior doctor. Let's have a think about planning the order that the patients should be seen in the morning following handover. There is a logical way of progressing around the five wards where these patients usually are, but life is not that easy. There are two sick patients who are deteriorating (not on the same ward of course). There is one patient definitely ready for discharge who needs a discharge letter writing and their 'drugs for home' (or TTOs) prescribing. You have already been bleeped by the bed manager to tell you that the delayed discharge of that patient is stopping another one being admitted who is about to breach the 4-hour wait target in the Emergency Department. The Consultant (Dr Harris) is rather set in their ways and always likes to do the ward round in the same order. What are you going to do?

OK—had a moment to think about it? Dr Harris has now arrived—what are you going to suggest as your plan?

There are of course a myriad of alternatives but we will consider a few.

Option 1
Say nothing; let Dr Harris take their usual route and risk the health of the two sick patients and have a late discharge and a breach in the Emergency Department.

Option 2
Explain the issues to Dr Harris and delegate 'up' so that the decision-making is done by the most senior member of the team. But you have concerns about the approachability of Dr Harris and you are not quite sure how to have the conversation. You put it off and only manage to broach the subject part way through the ward round.

Option 3
You explain the situation to the SHO/CT1 (Senior House Officer or equivalent, i.e. the next level of experience on the medical team) and/or the Registrar. They should have more experience in planning and prioritizing. They should also have developed their assertiveness skills when having to challenge a Consultant. The Registrar phones Dr Harris and asks to delay the ward round. Both the SHO and the Registrar go to a sick patient, whilst you are told to go and write the discharge letter and TTOs. You are then told to phone the bed manager and liaise with the ward Sister to get that patient to the discharge lounge. When

you finish that you are to join the SHO at the bedside of sick patient number 2. The ward round starts half an hour later than planned but everyone is safe and happy.

Option 4
You decide to ask for some advice from the Senior Sister on the ward round. She has worked with Dr Harris for years and is well versed in coping with her 'moods'. She suggests a pre-ward round briefing so that everyone is aware of the issues. Dr Harris surprises everyone and suggests a 'divide and conquer' approach similar to the one described in Option 3. Perhaps some of the pre-conceptions about Dr Harris were potentially going to cause a safety issue all on their own.

I will leave you to contemplate which option you prefer and what the long-term consequences of each might be. Life is not black and white and so I do not wish to present this in a way that there is only one clear right answer. Wouldn't that be easy!

Familiarity with our environments, or lack of, can play a role in error. It is important to understand our way around the hospital or departments or between hospitals. This needs to be included in the induction programme and should not be taken for granted early in a new post.

Static environment

I want you to consider the very basics of the environment in which you work. I will illustrate these factors with a few healthcare-based examples.

Atmospheric composition (air) and humidity

An example of the relevance of the air is the flow through an orthopaedic theatre where joint surgery may be taking place and the quality of that air is an essential component of trying to reduce infection. This may also be an important consideration if there has been a major disaster or a case of poisoning with certain chemicals.

Temperature

The temperature control mechanisms of a premature neonate have not yet matured and hence the environment must be tailor-made to optimize their care. In theatre it is often necessary to warm our patients and after a cardiac arrest there will be a group of patients that are cooled.

Be aware that the temperature may affect how well you are concentrating.

Smell

Have you ever walked on to a ward and been met by a smell? We need to do our very best to make the environments in which we care for our patients as pleasant as possible for our patients, their relatives, and our staff. Cleanliness needs to be a top priority as it is a basic human right.

I remember that a patient of mine who was feeling incredibly nauseous following her chemotherapy became very sensitive to smells. She found that the smell of perfume that one of the staff insisted on wearing was a real trigger for her vomiting!

Smells can of course, be useful to us to alert us of the presence of chemicals or gases (or the anaesthetic vapour that someone forgot to turn off!) or the cement that is being mixed ready for a joint replacement.

I once worked with a surgeon who was anticipating an unpleasant time whilst performing a manual evacuation of rectum who decided to insert a pre-injection swab up each nostril to disguise the smell and enable him to complete the task.

Lighting

It can be difficult to observe fine detail in dim light and also to interpret colour accurately. Consider whether this might be relevant to you.

I have only had to work on the roadside at a couple of emergencies but I take my hat off to those who have to work in suboptimal levels of lighting and temperature and environment in general.

I am almost trying to avoid the clichés about the anaesthetist adjusting the light for the surgeon in theatre but actually it is very important that they can see what they are doing.

In the same way as if you are using an instrument to view something inside a patient (endoscope, laparoscope, laryngoscope, etc.) the light source is vital and needs checking prior to insertion into the patient.

One of the most challenging environments I have worked in from a lighting perspective was in eye theatre when, for a particular procedure, it is necessary to function in darkness. There is a small amount of light from a light on the anaesthetic machine but it isn't possible to see the other staff. This means that all non-verbal communication is lost.

Noise levels

Continuing on with the theme of eye theatre, it became apparent to me early in my time in anaesthesia that the almost silent atmosphere in which some surgeons like to work was not going to blend well with my 'Tigger-like' personality.

We need to be acutely aware of the impact we are having on others' concentration levels and ability to function. If you are likely to have something to do that may need an increased level of cognitive demand, try and anticipate it. Explain to those around you at which stage you will need it to be quiet and why. This is best done first in a briefing before the whole episode commences and then it can be highlighted briefly when the time arrives without a long commentary.

In an emergency setting there is a tendency for people to lose the situational awareness of the part they are playing in the big picture. There are times when people talk over each and interrupt and they all want to talk at once. One of the roles of the good team leader is to channel this talking so that it happens in a logical sequence. Nobody talking in this setting is also a problem as there is no sharing of vital information.

There are many other noises around us apart from those generated by human voices. Despite what some surgeons tease you about, the noise from the monitor to tell you that the patient's heart is beating is essential. Not only can you subconsciously listen to the rate and rhythm of the heart beat but also the tonal change that accompanies a change in oxygen saturation is a noise with which all anaesthetists will be familiar. I think there is probably an inverse law about the tone of that monitor changing (as the oxygen levels in the patient drop and a serious situation is developing) and the rising heart rate of the anaesthetist (as their realization of events occurs).

While designing new equipment, it is necessary to consider the learnt behaviour that relies on taking cues from subconscious noises. Examples include the inflation of the blood pressure cuff and the noise that precedes it and the clunk of the old-fashioned ventilators.

There are noises that are not part of the safety process and in fact, at the other end of the scale, there are noise levels that can be hazardous. An example of the latter would be an MRI (magnetic resonance imaging) scanner. In this setting, it is important for both patients and staff to wear ear protection. Of note, are small anaesthetized children when I would recommend ear plugs which are taped in place in addition to the headphones.

We have already mentioned the lack of privacy and inadequate confidentiality that come into play with the assumption that curtains around bed-spaces are sound proof. The same applies for standing at a reception desk in a GP surgery or clinic or even at a pharmacy desk.

Size

The size of the environment, as I've already alluded to when discussing the size of a lift, can be very important. I have also had my moan about designing corridors and the width of doors but there are many more examples where the task to be performed has not been considered when at the design phase of the building. The size of our storage areas is also an area that needs to be planned more effectively.

The space around a bed is often inadequate when you have a team of people trying to resuscitate someone. Even worse, is if someone has collapsed in the toilet. I would like to make a plea for common sense to prevail over the use of some arbitrary red tape. In a life-threatening or urgent setting, we do not have the time to follow lengthy manual handling policies, we need to put our patient's safety as paramount, and there is no time for 'faffing'.

There are also some specialized environments whose size needs careful planning, for example, if trying to complete a task inside an incubator or the limited space inside the bore of a MRI scanner which some patients find claustrophobic (hence the creation of a more open version of the scanner that feels less closed in).

How much space do you have in your environment?

Security

We have spoken of the problem of arriving at another department or hospital with a sick patient, only to find that you cannot gain access as you do not have the correct swipe card or pass code.

There are, of course, the usual safety issues of only letting people follow you through a security door if you know who they are. We should all wear our ID (identification) badges. There have been security issues (fortunately rarely) with people impersonating staff. Although it saddens me to say it, there are also regular thefts from healthcare sites.

We also have vulnerable patients who need to stay with us for their own protection. The environments which constitute 'safe' for these individuals must also be considered. In these cases something as simple as a cot side may be important.

Factors to consider in safety-controlled environments

◆ Radiation (e.g. x-ray, radiotherapy, CT scanner)

◆ Electromagnetic field (e.g. MRI)

◆ Biochemical hazard (e.g. chemotherapy, decontamination)

◆ Other hazard (e.g. laser, proximity to oxygen supply).

Tidiness

The last one on this list, which was devised by healthcare workers themselves, is the tidiness of the environment. I think this is not only for the aesthetic that it makes a more pleasant environment for our patients, their relatives, and our staff, but also that it makes it easier to find everything. We will return to the latter when we start to consider organization and standardization of each area.

Environment—task-related design

Resource location

◆ Knowing where it is

◆ Visibility

◆ Accessible

◆ Organized

◆ Standardized

◆ Optimized.

Let us imagine that I arrive on a ward as I have been asked to come and put in a cannula (plastic drip tubing that goes into a vein). I don't know the ward. I usually work in theatre. I am helping someone as they have been unable to manage to complete the task. I have located the ward and introduced myself to the staff and I have asked where the cannulas are stored. I am directed to the store cupboard. I spend the next 10 minutes hunting about for only a few items. The items seem to be stored randomly in a number of different drawers. The drawers are unmarked and a couple of them are difficult to open as a couple of cardboard boxes have been left in the storeroom.

In my alternate reality the situation may be rather different. When I walk into the storeroom I am met with a scene where each drawer has a photo and a clear label displaying its contents. The labels are colour coded. The items are grouped according to the task for which they are needed. The system is standardized across all the wards so that I don't have to learn a new layout when I am called to a different ward. The storage area for cardboard boxes is away from the drawers so that I can easily access the drawers without having to move anything.

An alternative would be to be able to pick up a pack that had everything you needed in one go or a set of portable drawers that could go to the patient's bedside.

The same type of system would be needed for each regularly performed task, e.g. insertion of urinary catheter (tube that goes into the bladder).

All the items that are used regularly are in the storage cupboard that is close by. Only those items that are used infrequently are stored further away so it minimizes trips up and down the ward. Have you ever considered the distances covered by a nurse whose laundry store is at the far end of the ward?

If we return to my fantasy ward, imagine that there is a fantastic stock system that means as the items are running low everything is re-ordered but without having too much stock sitting there as it is 'dead money'.

I believe that the 'Productive' series attempts to introduce systems to make this type of thinking become a reality.

Your Environment

I would like you to spend a few minutes considering the layout of the environment(s) in which you work.

I want you to think about your **immediate vicinity, i.e. within arm's reach**. How is it laid out? Can you reach what you need to reach? Would it be more efficient if things were in a different place or different order? Can you see all the things you need to see without having to crane your neck or do an owl impression? Are the right things in your eyeline?

If you are setting up a sterile field for a procedure, is there continuity from the trolley to the part of the patient on which you will be working? Is it laid out logically for the order you will need things?

If you are working in anaesthetics, can you see your monitor and your patient and your surgeon without relying on the lie I was told as a child that grown-ups have eyes in the back of their heads? With my tongue removed from my cheek, can you stand facing the patient and the surgeon and still be able to scan the monitor without moving your head? Is the monitor adjustable in height so that you can move it into your eyeline depending on whether you are seated or standing?

As a laparoscopic surgeon have you considered the height of the table, the whereabouts of the screen and its height and its angle, and whether the scrub nurse and assistant can also see the screen and reach the table?

If you are working in an open-plan office, how are you going to manage your interruptions? Have you considered a visual cue system (flag or post it on the PC) to signify when you do not want to be disturbed? Are you going to have to invest in some headphones as a visual cue that you don't want to be interrupted by people just wandering up to your desk to ask you something?

When you are planning a meeting or an interview, how do you design the furniture layout? What about for a teaching session? And with a patient—how should the room be then? What about when you are with distressed relatives?

And then there is another pet hate of mine—the ward round.

I wish to digress to illustrate something, please try Exercise 4.1.

Exercise 4.1 Christmas

I want you to imagine that it is Christmas time. In a 'post turkey and a few glasses' type way at a typical family Christmas scene it is now time for the annual event—a game of charades. Aunty Doris has been very enthusiastic with her planning this year and has done handmade charades that are pre-prepared. She says they have an interesting twist. When your name is drawn out of the hat first, you take your charade out of the hat and open it. It explains that this year's charades will be emotions and behaviours. You have got to act out *'intimidation'*. Have a think for a minute, how are you going to demonstrate that non-verbally? Have you decided how to do it?

You approach your fantasy sibling in their reindeer jumper and enter their personal space. You use your height as you are standing and they are sitting so you can look down at them. You stare hard with an unrelenting gaze and intense eye contact. There is no smile.

With record speed, the guesses are correct.

And what has that got to do with a ward round?

When you go to bed tonight I want you to just pause for a couple of minutes. When you are in your night-time attire, sit for a moment with a couple of pillows behind you and pull on your bed covers. Now imagine that the ward round has just arrived at your bedside. If you have a spouse or a partner or a house-mate ask them to come and stand over you. Contemplate how safe you feel in the comfort of your own home and consider whether it might be different in a hospital bed?

I would like to share a personal example (see Example 4.3).

Change always works best if it is organic and grows from within rather than being imposed from external sources. Ideally, if you run ward rounds in this 'old-school' manner then it would be most likely to succeed if you decide on alternative methods yourself that would suit your team. It is thus a tailor-made solution. What is suggested in Example 4.5 is simply one of many solutions that may provide alternatives. Before we get to that, we need to examine what functions a ward round currently serves (see Example 4.4).

Example 4.3 I am the patient

I have had three children and two different types of surgery, one as an inpatient and another as a day case. I believe the experience of being a patient is invaluable for all hospital staff.

I would like you to consider how the ward might look from a hospital bed. I want you to imagine the patient's environment. What are the sights, noises, smells, privacy, and level of cleanliness that you can see from this bed? If you have time the next time you are at work go and sit on a bed and look around you.

There are two other perspectives I would like you to consider, one is being pushed along a corridor in your nightwear or a hospital gown. How would that feel?

And the final one is to lie on a trolley and look up at people in an anaesthetic room, an experience that changed my practice.

I would like to tell you about my own personal experience of a ward round. I was already a consultant at the time. I would consider myself to be fairly assertive. I had a list of questions that I wanted to ask. The consultant, a nurse, and two trainees arrived in my room. They seemed busy. No one was on my level. The questions I had were personal.

The combination of factors meant that I did not ask my questions. I simply offered up that everything was fine and smiled.

I reflected that the ward round wasn't even that big. I saw far bigger ward rounds walk past me every day. I had been part of enormous teaching rounds as a student. Why was this so far from a patient-centred approach? Who on earth came up with this idea and why? Why do we just accept it as an ingrained system?

What would have helped?

As a patient I needed to feel safe. I wanted to talk to one person or at the very most two, but really only one. I needed to feel that they had time for me. I needed them to be at my eye-level. I needed them to ask the right questions. I needed them to know how to listen. I needed them to know how to wait and use silence.

I have thought long and hard about this. This is what I've come up with so far (see Example 4.5).

We need a completely new approach to this model. This constitutes an enormous change of a system that is a staple part of the health service. All change is resisted. This will be an uphill struggle. It will be laughed at and lots of eyes will 'sky'. Like any change we will need enthusiastic early adopters who are willing to put their heads above the parapet. I hope that maybe you will be one?

Example 4.4 Ward round

Let us start by unpicking the functions of a ward round:

1. The first component is the business round. This should involve a review of the patient history, physical findings, investigation results, current and trending observations, drug and treatment review, culminating in the working diagnosis and management plan to date. This should include multi-professional input.

2. The teaching round. There is an opportunity to practise presenting patients and receive constructive feedback on not only the presenting skills themselves but also on the diagnostics and management plan. There is a role modelling or apprentice style chance to observe a senior clinician at work with regard to history, examination, critical thinking, team working, communication skills, prioritizing, and planning.

3. There is time for the team to function together and to potentially discuss any challenges that are faced and seek senior input. These may be either clinical challenges or logistical ones. A job list is created (who needs blood tests, surgery, a CT scan, to be discharged, a referral to another team, etc.). A management plan for each patient is decided.

4. But what about the patient? What would they like? Have you asked them (not in the middle of a ward round!)?

5. Perhaps there would be something about being listened to or able to ask questions? Perhaps something about confidentiality or privacy and dignity? Perhaps something about feeling there would be time? Maybe seeing the expert would feature? Perhaps the language that is used to explain tricky concepts would be expressed? Maybe they would want to have some honesty? Perhaps they would want to know what the long-term plans might be? Perhaps they don't want a huge herd of people staring down at them in their bed?

How will you find out what your patients think?

With all of that in mind, could you plan your ward round differently? What system could you use? How would you know whether the patients were happy? The latter doesn't involve asking them what they think as part of a ward round!

An alternative is presented in Example 4.5.

Example 4.5 A new approach to ward rounds?

Let us suppose that we can try a new system.

Instead of starting on the ward there is a briefing in either an office or teaching area or in a department.

The briefing takes the form of a handover in a set format with pre-prepared information in the form of an SBAR (situation, background, assessment, recommendation/request) handover sheet which is included here (but it is covered in much more detail later, see handover in Chapter 7).

This list is something that is built upon electronically (ideally) and is accessible from all clinical areas (first challenge for some, easy for others). If we were clever about using an electronic patient record, some of it could populate automatically.

Situation There is a description of the name, whereabouts and diagnosis of each patient.

Background A brief background of any salient points, including positive physical findings and investigation results.

Assessment A recent review of physiological parameters and an early warning scoring system.

Recommendations This should include the current management plan and a conversation about potential discharge date if relevant.

The briefing might go something along the lines of this:

Roles are allocated so that one person sits at a computer and it is their role to display blood results, chest x-rays or other films, and the most recent physiology or electronic record if there is that capability. The drug chart could also be reviewed if it is electronic.

Handover sheets are printed off for everyone who wants one (taking care that the information is handled sensitively and not left on the bus later!).

The senior person may scan the list and spot a high score on the physiological parameters of the early warning score and decide to deal with this now

---

(has outreach been triggered? Can we send one of the team to review this patient? Should I go myself?).

There is a logical presentation of each of the patients using the SBAR framework. There is ideally a double act here. Whilst one person is presenting, the other is on the computer displaying any relevant information as discussed.

There can still be teaching and business in this format. By standardizing the information flow (using SBAR) there is evidence that it is more accurate.

Feedback on performance and learning should become normal. There should be praise.

Once the briefing is completed, a decision can be made about the order of reviewing the patients.

On arriving on the ward (ideally in time slots so that all the ward rounds do not arrive at once!) there is a nurse allocated to join the round.

For each patient, there is an update by the nurse of anything that may have happened in the recent time frame.

The full ward round does not enter each bay! Perhaps the senior person (on their own) or perhaps the senior and the nurse or the senior and one trainee go to the bedside. They have an appropriate conversation giving attention to body language, eye levels, empathy, and time. There is time for the patient to ask questions and to be examined.

While this is happening the rest of the team are not idle. They review the patient's notes and drug chart. They discuss the diagnosis and they ask two important questions.

'What are we missing here?'

'What else could this be?'

These questions are asked every day. It is important to stop the answer becoming a reflex answer of 'nothing'. Perhaps each person in turn tries to name an alternative diagnosis or missing step in the treatment? Perhaps you try and anticipate—what could go wrong with this patient? Where is the next opportunity for an error here?

Do the relatives know what is happening?

When the bedside team return, the notes are updated. There is a mini debrief for that patient. Someone summarizes, someone writes or types. Information from the 'bedside team' and the 'preventing assumption/error spotting team' are shared. A plan is made (including potential discharge if applicable). Jobs to go onto the job list are allocated.

And repeat with each patient.

It shouldn't take any longer than the current methods as there are no rambling handovers or presentations, something structured and targeted and safer instead.

At the end of the round, there should be debrief and feedback. This should include targeted praise. There should be a summary of the jobs to be done and help with the decision-making of the planning and prioritizing. This can be tackled by asking questions (coaching style) rather than 'micromanagement' or pacesetting.

What are your thoughts?

Are you denying there is a problem? All my patients are happy. Are they?

Are you confused? Will it 'never work'? Is it all very well 'but just not right for your environment'? Is it someone else's decision?

Are you resisting a change? If so, why is that?

Or might you give it a go? Play with it? Make it your own? Delight in tailor-making it to make your patient's experience improve and to make the information transfer more complete and reduce fixation and assumption?

Key points from Chapters 1–4

◆ We all make mistakes. Are you looking at how to avoid your next one?

◆ We need to embed an open culture. Culture is one of many informal systems in which we function.

◆ There should be an inquisitive approach to error that seeks out the learning and shares it: the learning culture.

◆ This should include 'memory checks' and 'safety events'.

◆ The new error checklist—the SHEEP sheet—helps gather more information following an actual event or a nearly event. It is quick and easy to use.

◆ The SHEEP sheet can be used for trend analysis.

◆ Information flow across an organization can be achieved using a brief/debrief model using Debbie's Diamond.

- Systems errors are commonly part of the holes in the Swiss cheese model and should feature in the solutions for improved safety.

- Things are not always what they seem: avoid assumption.

- 'What am I missing here?' is a healthy question to keep asking.

- If the hierarchy is too steep, the team will not feel able to challenge the leader when they are making a mistake. We all make mistakes.

- If there is a flat hierarchy, no natural leader emerges—ask the question, 'Who's leading?'

- Followership is a much overlooked and important skill to have. This can involve being assertive enough to speak up if things are about to go wrong.

- We will all push someone else's buttons. We can't change the other person, only ourselves.

- We need to become more aware of how we are impacting on others (increase our self-awareness). This might begin with knowing our preferred learning style, team role, and our personality type (MBTI).

- Once we know who we are more likely to 'clash' with, we can try and blend in a bit better (self-management) to avoid conflict.

- If we do end up in conflict we will behave in an assertive way (this is completely different from aggressive although the terms are often misused) and aim to find a win–win situation.

- A good leader will be able to switch to using four different leaderships styles when appropriate and will avoid micro-management or pacesetting. (This pacesetting style currently dominates the NHS in both clinical and non-clinical leaders.)

- Remember when giving feedback and praise:

  Situation Behaviour Impact Change or Continue.

- Knowing where everything is and having it laid out in a logical clearly marked way not only makes it more efficient but it makes it safer.

- Standardizing clinical areas decreases errors.

- If you are doing a transfer, plan and plan some more. Have a plan A, B, C, D in case it all goes wrong.

- Interruptions are huge problems in healthcare. Try not to interrupt others. If you are interrupted yourself, start the task again if you can and watch for errors.

- Try not to stand over patients in their beds and talk down to them. Always imagine how they might be feeling.

- SBAR—situation, background, assessment, recommendation/request—is good for handovers of information especially on the phone.

5

The second 'E' of SHEEP: Equipment

As busy brains must beat on tickle toys,
As rash invention breeds a raw device,
So sudden falls do hinder hasty joys:
And as swift baits do fleetest fish entice,
So haste makes waste

George Gascoigne (1534–77)
No haste but good (1573)

I'm not sure that one will appeal to all, so I'm including an alternative for this chapter:

Man is a tool making animal

Benjamin Franklin (1706–1790)
James Boswell, *Life of Samuel Johnson* (1791), 7 April 1778

Introduction

Let's start by exploring the second 'E' of the algorithm (see Figure 5.1). To clarify, we use the word 'equipment' to cover the wide range of objects with which we interact. Some of these are inanimate objects (such as a sterile drape) that serve a purpose but we don't really interact with them. Some are tools (such as a scalpel or laparoscope) which we use to complete a task. Another group are machines with which we interact (physiological monitor or computer). Other groups of materials have also been included: drugs, blood products, and prostheses.

I will tackle this section in three broad categories: generic equipment issues, user–equipment interface issues, and then much more specific equipment issues. I will illustrate each section with examples of real errors (fully anonymous, of course.). This chapter is more relevant to those of you with a clinical

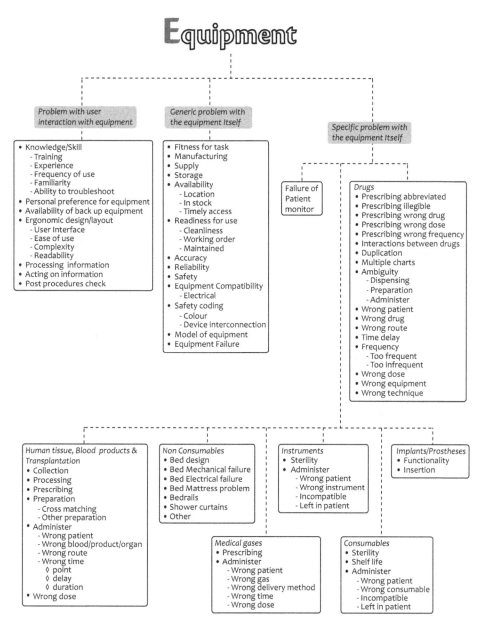

Figure 5.1 'E'—the SHEEP model.

role but for those of you who are non-clinical it is useful to understand the challenges that are faced by your colleagues.

The first thing to consider is the design of the equipment. Whilst most of the equipment design occurs before we have anything to do with it, we need to influence manufacturers so that we have a say in how our equipment is designed.

You may well have considered in what position you like your car seat in terms of both how far away you are from the pedals and the angle of the seat. And how you like your mirrors adjusted to optimize your view. You may have adjusted the height of your steering wheel. You may prefer the layout of one dashboard over another or the indicator to be one side and the wipers on the other. I wonder why car manufacturers have not standardized these designs.

You may also have considered how high you like your desk chair, whether you prefer a keyboard with or without a tilt, and whether you like your computer screen close to you or further away. You may have gone as far as to consider the angle of your arms when typing. You may have a preference for the feel of a particular set of keys when typing or you may be developing a preference for a touch screen. What will influence how much time you have spent thinking about it? Perhaps if working with a computer constitutes a greater proportion of your job this may be an influencing factor?

You may be aware that cash point machines were redesigned so that they give you your card back before your cash to try to stop you leaving the card behind.

Another commonly used example about equipment design in everyday use is a cooker hob. If we consider that there are four rings on a hob laid out in a two-by-two square, what would be the optimum way of displaying the controls so that it is obvious which control operates which ring? (See Figure 5.2.)

Figure 5.2 shows two diagrams of four ring hobs with a control for each ring. With the first example the control panel is displayed in a way that leaves some

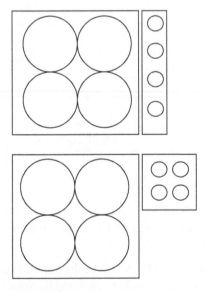

Figure 5.2 Four ring hobs.

ambiguity over which dial operates which ring. In the second example, it is completely clear which dial operates which ring.

How much time have you spent considering the design of other equipment that you interact with?

Considerable thought has gone into making anaesthetic machines safer over the years. I will run through some of the safety features of an anaesthetic machine to illustrate some of the ideas that have been incorporated to serve as an example (see Example 5.1)

Example 5.1 The anaesthetic machine

A simple review of some of the safety features on an anaesthetic machine (examples only, not an exhaustive list, nor a complete exam answer!). Also included is a word of caution about how modernizing machines may cause safety issues.

There are different pipes which supply different gases into an anaesthetic machine (currently three: oxygen, air, and nitrous oxide). They are colour coded to make it easy to identify which one is for each gas. At the end of the pipe is a special fitting that has a unique shape for each gas and will only fit into the complementary fitting in the wall that is for the same gas.

The colour coding continues on the front of the machine with standardized colours for gases and anaesthetic agents.

The knobs that exist on older machines to turn on the gases were not only colour coded but also had different shapes and the oxygen was set so that it stuck out more from the machine. A lot of these safety features have been lost when we have modernized and switched to digital displays.

The older generation of anaesthetists (me included) were used to watching a bobbin spinning within a glass tube which was a visual cue that gas was flowing. The identification of this reliance on a visual cue led to a split in designs when the newer era of anaesthetic machines were introduced. Some manufacturers opted for a digital display that represented the glass tubes, whilst others decided to simply replace it with a numerical display.

It is vitally important to consider how information is gathered and processed.

I had an interesting discussion with Roger Kneebone following a keynote speech he gave. He suggested that the surgeon at an operating table had in front of them the equivalent of a cone, which represented the zone of visual field focus. I have no quibbles about this. My levels of interest rose when he assumed that the anaesthetist was the same and in fact he assumed that the focus would be on the head of the patient. Whilst this may be the case at the very beginning of the case when instrumenting the airway (putting a device in someone's mouth in most cases), this is not the case once they are on the operating table. He challenged me, that if I didn't like his analogy, I should come up with my own, so here it is. I think we need three cones.

Cone 1

If we imagine a time in the middle of a longer case that is progressing in a routine manner, where might our eyes be looking? I think there is a focused cone but that it moves between the monitor on the anaesthetic machine (where I suspect it spends a good proportion of its time) and the patient and the records we are writing. Perhaps it doesn't move with the regularity of a windscreen wiper or a game at Wimbledon but is regularly changing.

Within that cone I think each experienced anaesthetist develops a way of scanning the mixture of waveforms and digital data to glean the information required.

Cone 2

I think we also need a wider cone to maintain good situational awareness. If our zone of focus is on the monitor, with our wide cone we can still absorb what the surgeon and scrub nurse and anaesthetic assistant are doing. It is important to be aware whether things are progressing to plan or are becoming more challenging or whether it won't be long until we finish and so it's time to send for the next patient.

Cone 3

The 'third cone equivalent' is not a visual one but an auditory one. I wonder whether a lighthouse is a suitable analogy for the third cone. If instead of a light you imagine the beam to represent an absorption of sound waves.

We are subconsciously listening for sounds from the monitor. The 'beep beep' noise gives us the rate and rhythm of the heart beat and the tone gives us the oxygen saturation level. The older ventilators made a noise, as did the older style blood pressure cuffs that signalled to us subconsciously that those activities were taking place.

In addition, we can hear a noise from the partially obstructed airway of the patient or the suction bottle filling with blood. We can hear a change in the tone of voice of the surgeon as the stress levels are rising following a problem. Or perhaps keep track of a more routine conversation about what happened at the weekend.

We may also be teaching simultaneously.

This presents a very high cognitive workload for those of us who were traditionally considered to be just doing a crossword!

Returning to the anaesthetic machine, there are spare gas cylinders on the back of the machine in case the pipeline gases fail. There is a mechanism that prevents delivery of a hypoxic mixture (stops you giving too little oxygen by mistake). There is an Ambu bag on the back of each anaesthetic machine in case the whole machine fails and you need to ventilate by hand.

The anaesthetic agents themselves are in colour coded bottles (isoflurane is purple, sevoflurane is yellow, halothane used to be red, and yes, I am that old!). There is an attachment on the top of the bottle which is put on when you wish to put the volatile (anaesthetic drug) into the vaporizer (a special bit of the machine which is also colour coded which is where the anaesthetic is stored). There is an interlocking mechanism on the neck of the bottle that again only allows the correct attachment for that volatile. On the top end of the attachment there is a different shape 'key' which only fits into the right vaporizer.

The idea is that no matter how stressful the circumstances when you are trying to refill a vaporizer with anaesthetic, it is almost impossible to mix up the wrong drug.

This is not an exhaustive list of all of the safety features. I have chosen a mixture to illustrate some different ideas.

The idea of interlocking connections is to be adapted to make giving drugs intrathecally (into the spinal fluid in your back) safer. Only those drugs that are intended to go into spinal fluid will have the right attachment on the end of their syringe. This will hopefully very much reduce the chances of the wrong chemotherapy drug being injected into the wrong place (i.e. the drug that should be given into the vein will no longer be able to be given into the spinal fluid as it will not be possible to attach the syringe in which it is contained to the spinal needle).

I wonder also whether it might be possible to draw inspiration from this device in car manufacturing. Would it be possible to shape the nozzles at a fuel pump so that a diesel pump could only interlock with the cap on a car that takes diesel? This would potentially eliminate the whole wrong fuel wrong car scenario. I will leave you to ponder why I am contemplating this particular scenario. I digress.

I want you to consider for a moment any equipment that you work with. If you have time make a written list of all of the machines and tools. How familiar are you with any safety features? Do you know anything about the design of the equipment? Should you know? How could you find out more? How could you influence the future design of safety features? If you find yourself saying, 'I wish it could just do . . . ' or 'it would be better if . . . ', have you spoken to someone about your idea? Is it fit for purpose?

After the design phase is the manufacturing. Might there be a relevant step in any of the equipment or tools or machines or drugs or blood products or implants or consumables with which you are involved where a manufacturing fault might be important? How would you know there was one? What checks are in place to try and prevent it from having a significant impact on patient care? Do you know what checks the equipment should have been through? Or is that simply 'someone else's problem'? If so, who is 'someone' and how do you know they have done their job?

There are not infrequent episodes in industry of devices being recalled. In the last year I can think of a model of car, a pram, and a make of soft drink that were all recalled due to manufacturing errors. How would you know you had one? What would you do about it? How might you hear if something had been withdrawn or had an alert about it? How would you ensure this information was cascaded appropriately?

There has been a manufacturing issue with one of the anaesthetic drugs over a year ago. This led us to have to change the technique that is used for emergency anaesthetics. We had to adjust to using a different agent that behaves quite differently (it has a slower, less predictable onset). This involved modifying the whole technique. This change in supply came without much warning and the training that needed to be delivered to staff had to be delivered in a short time frame. I admit to having misjudged one of my early cases using the new technique when I expected the patient to be asleep and found that they were still talking to me!

The storage of surgical instruments, drugs, and blood products will be used to illustrate a few examples of how the storage itself can be an issue (see Examples 5.2–5.4). They also show the importance of availability with particular reference to location and timely access.

Example 5.2 Orthopaedic theatre

A busy orthopaedic list is already underway. The morning began with a thorough briefing (using the WHO checklist) and it was highlighted that one of the sets was still to arrive from the place where it is sterilized. The first two cases which were knee arthroscopies have gone very efficiently and the set has arrived just in time. The porter has gone to collect the next patient.

When the scrub nurse starts to open the set to prepare for the next case she identifies a hole in the wrapping of the set. She stops what she is doing and comes to talk to the surgeon. In the meantime the patient has just arrived in the anaesthetic room. In amongst the preoperative checks the patient expresses extreme relief at finally having their joint surgery. They share how difficult it has been to arrange care for an elderly relative and how the time has been booked off from work and how much rescheduling that took. The anaesthetist is about to insert a cannula when the scrub nurse asks if they could just have a word.

There is a multi-professional conversation about the breach in the sterility of the instruments and the possible alternatives. Fortunately the team reach a creative solution that means that rather than cancel the case completely, the patient can be moved to last on the list allowing turnaround of another surgical set.

Example 5.3 Blood storage

There is a pregnant lady who is losing a lot of blood who has been admitted to the Emergency Department at 18 weeks (out of a normal 40 weeks of a full-term pregnancy). Her records reveal that she has a rare blood grouping and antibodies that means that the usual backup blood group (O-negative) is not suitable for her. The only blood that is suitable for her is in the regional hospital. It will take at least 45 minutes by even the fastest of blue light transport to bring it and that is once it has been issued. The total estimated time will be close to 1 hour and 30 minutes. Like many young people the woman has physiologically compensated well, but she is suddenly decompensating. Her blood pressure is dropping fast and her conscious level has now dropped. The surgeon wants to take her to theatre now. She is in desperate need of blood products. The haemoglobin result shows a level of 3.4 (a normal result, even in pregnancy would be over 10) and this is life threatening.

Not all rare blood groupings can be stored in all places.

Example 5.4 Anaesthetic room

Some anaesthetic drugs need to be stored in the fridge or they start to become inactive. The morning list had been quite hectic as there had been an unexpected emergency. The muscle relaxant ampoules are contained in a box. In the hurry the whole box had been taken out of the fridge and left on the side. The individual had meant to put it away but was interrupted. Someone places some notes on the side and in the process, pushes the box so that it is now hidden behind some other items. It is now fulfilling the old cliché 'out of sight, out of mind'. By the time the workload finally settles, there has been a shift change of anaesthetic assistant. They are tidying the work surface and put the drug box back in the fridge. They have no idea that it has actually been sat there for almost 10 hours.

The problem does not become apparent until the following day. There are no visual cues that the drug is no longer as active. The drug is drawn up by a different group of staff who know nothing about what went on the previous day. No one knows there is a problem until there is a failure of the muscle relaxant to work.

Readiness for use

I have, on occasion, pulled out a piece of equipment from the storage area only to find that it is covered in blood and that the last person who put it away did not clean it! Along the same lines are when you go to use something, only to find that it is broken. We need to report faults and seek alternative solutions. We need to communicate to those whom this may affect that the problem has occurred and how long it will take to rectify. We need to think about the maintenance consequences of all equipment that we procure. Who will fund the maintenance? Who will perform it? What does the schedule for the frequency of the maintenance need to look like and what affect will this have on service provision? Is there an optimum time that would have least impact?

Let us next consider the concept of accuracy (see Example 5.5).

Example 5.5 Accuracy

It became apparent that the readings taken on different thermometers which were traditionally used at different stages of the perioperative period were giving very different readings. The ward staff were using a digital thermometer under the tongue (in a plastic sleeve). In theatre the anaesthetist was using an oesophageal or naso-pharyngeal temperature probe (no standardization as to position of probe placement). In recovery, the staff were using tympanic thermometers (nozzle placed in the ear and it beeps when it is finished). It was observed, by chance initially and later by audit, that there seemed to be a large discrepancy between the devices. After doing some background research as to establishing which should be the gold standard, the methods were standardized and the accuracy was assessed. There was then a decision to stop using the tympanic method. Although it was the least invasive method, the accuracy was not adequate for the task.

Reliability

Not only do we need our equipment to pass the 'Ronseal test', i.e. 'it does what it says on the tin', we need to do it every time, the same, without variation, and without failure.

If we consider a pump (broadly speaking this is an electronic device, smaller than a laptop, that pushes a syringe of drug continuously at a rate which can be decided) in the intensive care setting. There are two drugs being delivered via pump. One is a drug that keeps the patient sedated (sleepy enough to cope with the treatments) and the other is a drug that keeps blood pressure up to an adequate level. Not only do we want to know that if we ask the pump to deliver at 5mL per hour that is what it will do. We want to know it will do it over a pro-longed time frame, without giving too much or too little, and without stopping. If it stops delivering the sedation medicine, the patient may wake up and pull out some of their tubes which could be dangerous. If it stopped giving the medicine that maintains the blood pressure the blood pressure may drop, which in broad terms means not enough oxygen may be being delivered to vital organs such as the brain or the heart. Something equally detrimental would be if the pump stopped and then started again suddenly giving a bit extra of this blood pressure medicine. If the blood pressure suddenly shot up to a very high level this could potentially cause a stroke or in other settings may cause the patient to bleed.

If we consider a simpler device, a laryngoscope, what would a problem with reliability look like? (This is an instrument that is usually made of metal. It has two parts; a handle and a blade. In the handle bit, which as the name suggests you hold, there are traditionally some batteries which power a light source on the other bit—the blade. The blade is placed in a patient's mouth when they are asleep to move the tongue and adjust the angle of things so that the anaesthetist can see down the wind pipe where they want to put a tube. This is the process of intubation. The two parts of the instrument are attached together in a sort of hinge. The device has a resting state when the blade and the handle are next to each other. When the hinge is moved to bring the two parts closer to a 90-degree angle, they click into place. The light should activate at this point.) Let us consider the role of the light. The light should come on automatically when the instrument is moved to the 90-degree position. It is checked prior to the patient being put to sleep. There are times, however, when these devices have an intermittent fault. The anaesthetist has inserted the blade into the mouth and perhaps struggled to get a good view of the hole and just at that moment, the light fails! This can involve starting the process all over again. In a routine setting this may be of little consequence other than inconvenience and taking more time. In an emergency, when the patient is paralysed, the oxygen levels are dropping, and there is only a short time to get the tube in the hole, it can be dangerous for the patient and grey-hair inducing for the anaesthetist. It is paramount to always have a spare laryngoscope not just 'around' but within arm's reach.

Not all of the equipment that we interact with is clinical. Some of you may be able to relate to my next example more readily. On an office-based day, I have taken to arriving early. I hope the reason will become apparent. My first task is to turn on my computer. I then need to go and make a coffee. By the time I return my computer is just about ready to wake up. I have with time decided, with tongue firmly in check and scientific brain abandoned, that just like me, it seems to have good and bad days. I have begun to think of it of having a persona. I talk to it. I confess I am sometimes not polite to it. In terms of fitness for task, I have my doubts. As far as reliability is concerned, I wonder whether my tendency to consider it to more strongly resemble a human than a machine speaks for itself.

Safety of equipment

There are checks also on other sources of safety of the machines. The first example is the tragic example of Beth Bowen whose story is available from <http://www.patientstories.org.uk>.

A piece of equipment which was fully safe for a specified task (hysterectomy surgery) was used for something different from which it was designed (splenectomy) with the catastrophic result of the death of a young life.

Has the tool been designed for this purpose is a good self-check to be asking.

Have all the electrical checks been performed? There is something called microshock which can happen in a clinical setting. Because we put tubes into veins that go down into the heart, there is potential for a tiny amount of electricity to travel down these tubes and travel straight to the heart with potentially dire consequences. Precautions need to be taken at the design phase to try to avoid this eventuality.

Have the maintenance checks been carried out? Are the correct stickers displayed to confirm the last dates of these checks or is there a different system?

Let us consider some safety issues about the MRI machine. Not only are there the effects related to moving something that is metal, there can also be a heating effect of certain objects. It is so important to know if your patient has a pacemaker or a metal clip in their brain after surgery or a new joint replacement or some new clips on their tubes to stop them conceiving!

Multiple models of the equipment

When I began anaesthetics in one hospital about 17 years ago, every theatre had a different model of anaesthetic machine. They had been bought at different times and by different people who had their favourite machine (or favourite sales rep, yes, old and cynical!) This meant I was regularly facing the challenge of using a new machine that I had never seen before and had received no training on. Whilst I agree they were considerably simpler than they are now, they were very different. If any of you fancy a bit of history look up a Blease, a Manley, and a Penlon and see if you can work out what to do with them with no training! I found it a challenge.

The standardization of equipment models is vital. If there are historically still multiple versions around, training on the nuances of each version is essential. A business plan for their replacement should be implemented as soon as possible and could include the patient safety issues. I am not in favour of the attitude, we've been using these for years and nothing has happened . . . ! The next error could be just around the corner.

Equipment failure

In broad terms this could involve a failure that happens before you want to use an item, whilst you are using it, or it could be an intermittent fault or something that is gradually happening over time and you are not yet aware. Whilst it is frustrating to get equipment out of the storage facility only to discover that it is not working, at least you know where you stand before you start a procedure. It the failure happens right in the middle of something it can have far more consequences.

We could also classify our failure by other means, perhaps the type of failure: electrical, mechanical, physical, chemical, technical, environmental, or other.

Whatever the mode of the failure or when it occurs we need to plan and prepare for it.

For some of the simplest settings, we can have a spare one standing by and perform a substitution. Do you know where your spares are? Are you religious about checking they are there? Do you personally always check them? If you don't, then who does and how do you know they have done it? Do you at least have a conversation about it? Would it be worth incorporating it into a checklist?

The next option is to substitute it with something slightly different. I want you to ask yourself in that setting whether your decision is the best for your patient.

I would like you to locate both the SHEEP sheet (a copy of which is in the Appendix) and Example 5.6: Equipment failure. I admit the clue is in the title! I would like you to try and use the SHEEP sheet as you go along with the next scenario. After each sentence I would like you to ask yourself the following questions:

◆   Are there any factors that are present on the SHEEP sheet?

◆   How might each of those factors contribute to an error?

◆   What might that error be?

◆   How could I prevent it from happening?

This is a true story (see Example 5.6).

Example 5.6 Equipment failure

It was night time. The Intensive Care Unit (ICU) was full to overflowing. This has necessitated the use of a clinical area that is usually used for a different purpose to be used as an overflow ICU. It was unfamiliar. It was isolated from other departments. There were two nurses and two patients. There was no one to relieve them for breaks. Both staff were senior and experienced and diligent. There was no piped gas and so the ventilators were being run from cylinders. This means they needed to be changed periodically. There is no warning system to tell you the cylinder is running low. There is a visual gauge that indicates when the cylinder is low. Ventilators need a power supply to run. Monitors are the machine that has the screen that makes the beep noise and shows you the heart tracing, blood pressure tracing, oxygen level tracing, and so on. Monitors need electricity to run, although some of them may have a battery backup for a short amount of time. If a ventilator fails it is necessary to squeeze a special bag by hand to breath for the patient to keep them alive. This special bag should be stored with every ventilator. It often hangs on the back of the ventilator in a clear plastic bag. There should also be a piece of tubing that attaches the bag to the oxygen supply. At the beginning of every shift, the special bag should be checked. The wall phone had broken and so a temporary replacement had been placed on the desk. It had a mobile handset but the handset seemed to have a fault so that it could not hold any charge. Part way through the shift it stopped working altogether. Hospitals usually have a backup generator.

Here it comes.

There was a power cut. The emergency backup generator failed.

The room was pitch black. The ventilators stopped working. The nurses remained calm and went to the back of the ventilators (not as easy as it sounds in the dark when ICU patients have wires and tubes everywhere). They each located their bags but it was tricky to remove them from the bag in the dark. By feel, they located the tubes in the patient's mouths and attached the bags. They ventilated the patients by squeezing the bags by hand. Usually when you carry out this activity, you watch the rise and fall of the patient's chest to know how hard to squeeze the bag. They could not see the patient's chest! They therefore had one hand squeezing the self-inflating and the other on the patient's chest for the first few breaths until they were sure it was rising. The pair of nurses continued dialogue throughout. They encouraged and supported each other through every stage. Even if they had called for help, no one would have heard them. The monitors came back on as their own batteries seemed to kick in. Each of these batteries would have a finite life. This allowed a tiny amount of light. The tiny amount of light enabled them to see just enough to find the tubing from the bag and attach it from the self-inflating bag to the oxygen supply (a small cylinder that they each had standing by just in case!). Neither of these cylinders of oxygen would last very long. There were no spares in this area. Once the oxygen levels of each patient had stabilized they carefully planned their next steps.

One nurse managed to ventilate both patients intermittently for the brief period it took the other to cross the room, grab their handbag and return to the bedside. They found their mobile phone and contacted the site manager. The site manager came down, took over hand ventilating a patient, freeing up one of the nurses to make arrangements for more oxygen cylinders to be collected by the porters and various other plans to make the situation safe (light source, spare monitors, spare cylinders, communication system, regular checks by site manager, spare pumps). Both theatre and the main ICU were facing similar problems and so had no one spare to help. After what felt like the longest night shift ever, the power was restored at around dawn.

I think the nurses deserve a medal, but how often do we see our healthcare staff in an honours list? And of course, that is not why they do it, but a bit of public praise wouldn't go a miss.

Do you know what backups you need if you have a failure? Do you know where they are or how to mobilize them? Have you practised for these failures (for example, in a simulator)?

Workarounds following equipment failure or malfunction

I wanted to share a simple example of an equipment malfunction, a workaround, and a resultant error. It happened to me at lunchtime today and it made me smile. I am struggling a little with the usual seasonal affliction of having gained a few pounds over the festive period. Despite this I succumbed and ordered some 'thrice-cooked' chips with my lunch. I rather like my chips with ketchup and this is where the problem began. The ketchup was served in a dispenser with a spout but the spout seemed to be blocked. I tried the usual answers to equipment failures—I hit it, I started all over again, I shook it, I muttered under my breath, and I tried brute force, but to no avail. I decided to remove the top (my workaround). I had not anticipated the speed with which the ketchup would now arrive and the error that resulted was a veritable swimming pool of red in which my chips were now submerged. There were smiles and amusement, but no harm done. The clinical consequences of bending the rules, however, are not always positive.

So far we have looked at problems with the equipment itself. Of course, the equipment is not the only source of error. How we interact with the equipment can be the cause of some of the problems.

User–equipment interface

Before we use most types of equipment, we should be trained how to use it. (I admit you may not need to be trained on something very simple or commonplace.) The training should be of an adequate standard and repeated at an appropriate frequency. The latter will be influenced by a number of factors including the experience level of the individual, the frequency with which they use the equipment, and their familiarity with it. What level of training do you need? Do you simply need to be able to interact with the equipment, or if it failed, would you need to be able to troubleshoot to solve the problem?

We also need to know who needs what training, whether they have had it, and whether they will need it again, and if so, how often. Do you have a system in place for this? How accurate is it?

It may be worth you mulling over for a moment the equipment that you work with. Is there something that you use less frequently? Is there something that is relatively new? How will you ensure you are maintaining an adequate skill level?

Personal preference for equipment

Have you ever thought about what contributory factors there might be for your personal preferences for equipment?

If I ask you to consider buying a fantasy car in your head right now, take 1 minute to make a choice. What influences what car you have chosen? Are you considering the make or model or colour or reputation or reliability or safety or economy or 'green' or practicalities of a family and a dog or cost or speed or image or how does it handle? Are you thinking about whether it has a cup holder or heated seats or a tow bar or a curry hook or a sunroof or is it a convertible or a bike rack or roof bars?

If you are not a driver, perhaps consider the exercise with choosing a mobile phone or purchasing a laptop or a new computer: what would you choose and why?

If we bring these choices back to the workplace, one of the most current influencing factors is the financial constraints within which we must function. Every purchase we make means that something else is not purchased. I know that a number of my clinical colleagues are not taking adequate responsibility for their purchases. The argument put forward is that 'I want the best for my patient', which of course is what we all want. However, we have to think about all of the pieces of jigsaw. How can I say that my piece is more important than the other 499 pieces of the puzzle?

And so we find ourselves in a position of rationing and prioritizing. I find myself pondering a quote about the 'needs of the many over the needs of the few' and wondering how we should be making these difficult decisions. My request to the clinicians is not to be enticed by the latest fancy technological advance without thinking about the impact it will have on all of the patients within the organization.

Back to what it is that is important to us in decision-making with regards to equipment choice.

We will consider as an example the ergonomic design/layout of a monitor screen. The information displayed includes waveforms and digital data. When we start to think about a monitor, the first thing is that we need to be able to read it. This involves it being at an appropriate height, which might need to be adjustable. The screen needs not to be too reflective so that we can see it from different angles in differing light conditions and an auto-lit option for low lighting levels would be useful. The data must be displayed in a way that is not ambiguous. It must be clear which numerical value is associated with each variable. The numerics should be big enough and in an easy-to-read font. Care should be taken with regard to colour blindness. My personal belief is that there should be an international standard colour coding system for each waveform and numeric. I would prefer a touch sensitive screen and I would like to be able to enlarge it in an 'apple-esk' way. I would like it to be completely intuitive. I want the screen to be big enough so that I can see a long stretch of the waveform as this is the only way to see patterns of rhythms. I would like it to be impossible to disable the alarm system but I would like the alarm system to be accurate and well designed. I would like a silence button that lasts for 1 minute.

When considering equipment in a more generic way we need to consider the layout, the user interface, the ease of use versus the complexity of functions, and the readability as a bare minimum. We need to consider where our eyeline will be and what we might need to touch or hold and therefore what shape it might need to be. There are experts in ergonomics who should be involved at the design phase of all equipment but it is up to those who use it to communicate our needs.

Processing information

In order to process and assimilate information we must first perceive it. We are absorbing sensory information via our most basic of senses but the information is far from basic, it is very complex.

A theatre example is used to illustrate different ways that we perceive and then process information.

Visually from a monitor we can observe multiple waveforms and digital data. We are not just looking at single data points but we can pick up trends (e.g. a gradual lowering of the blood pressure over the last three readings taken at 2.5-minute intervals). Within the waveforms we can identify a change in rhythm on an ECG or when the muscle relaxant has worn off and the patient has started to breathe again simply by looking at the pattern of the carbon dioxide they are breathing out. These are each complex entities in their own right but we are looking at between four and six waveforms all the time and sometimes a great deal more. In addition, we are visually absorbing information from the patient themselves, for example, a change in skin colour may show us crude oxygen levels or a drop in haemoglobin levels (the red cells in blood which would go down if there was bleeding). We are also observing the surgeon and the procedure and the other members of the team and maybe the time. The subtlety of the body language that gives away whether the staff are working well together. Whether equipment preferences or failures are influencing how the day is unfolding, will all be taken in subconsciously.

Into this melee, we now add in some auditory stimuli. These may include the beep of the machine, the nuances of the tone of voice of those interacting in the room, the content of the conversation (social if things are progressing well and suddenly tense and focused clinically if they are not), a checklist, some teaching, a conversation about the next patient on the list, a bleep, a telephone, the suction filling with blood, an alarm alerting you to the drop in blood pressure, and perhaps some music in the background.

By meshing that information together we are starting to have a higher cognitive workload. These are not isolated sights and sounds but a complex monitoring system that is far beyond the capability of any computer. And that is before we taken in the smells (diathermy produces a fairly unique one) or the touch.

Basic clinical skills require an ability to feel lumps and bumps and identify size, consistency, and try to identify which plane they may be in. There are far more complex types of 'feel' or proprioception (knowing where bits of your body are) required. The feedback from a needle as it travels through different layers of skin and ligaments requires a different sort of processing altogether. What is being physically experienced must simultaneously be linked with a mental model of the anatomical layers through which the needle is travelling to try and find the right spot. This can require the cognitive ability to think in three dimensions, something which not everyone is skilled in and can be difficult to learn.

To cover the differences in processing between automatic versus conscious thought would take a chapter all by itself. For those of you who drive, have you ever arrived somewhere and not really remembered how you got there? It is possible when we are performing a task regularly for it to become routine so that we can complete it on autopilot and no longer have to concentrate on it. The fact that we are not concentrating on it, can, of course, cause problems. I would recommend that when you are tired or stressed that you make a conscious effort to switch out of automatic and try to concentrate as you are more likely to make a mistake at this time.

Acting on information

Yesterday, I had a problem with my home computer. It seemed that there may have been either a driver problem or maybe a threat from a virus. An 'autofix' mode that I had never seen before started itself. I found myself in a state of paranoia. Did such a mode exist or was it all really a virus? Today my laptop seemed to be making decisions all on its own and instead of behaving rationally and realizing the problem was in connection with my tracking function, I was instantly suspicious. The user interface in this case was not a logical one. It was coloured by my negative experience the previous day. I behaved irrationally and I could not troubleshoot what should have been relatively straightforward.

Why am I bothering to share this with you? There is a principle that underlies this story that seems to feature not infrequently in errors.

If an alarm on an anaesthetic machine goes off regularly when there is nothing wrong, it can become a 'crying wolf' phenomenon. If this inaccurate alarm becomes annoying enough and distracting enough, it may be that the individual will simply disable the alarm. Not only may that action impact on the current patient's care, but possibly on subsequent patients too. If the next clinician does not know the alarm has been disabled and is used to relying on it, this may have a knock-on effect. We need to improve the design of the equipment so that the false errors are minimized and so that the alarms cannot be disabled completely, only suspended for a standard amount of time.

If the blood pressure cuff seems to not be picking up a blood pressure, often the first action is to change the blood pressure cuff itself or to try and reposition it. The realities of a faulty or poorly positioned cuff are more palatable than the possible truth that the blood pressure may be very low. The actual sequence of action should be to check the patient clinically first as if the drop in blood pressure is the truth, then action should be taken promptly. We need to unlearn certain patterns of behaviour and replace them with new responses.

The warning system for low petrol used to be that the indicator on the gauge was in the red zone with the possible addition of a light coming on on the dashboard. In some models there is now an auditory beep to accompany the light turning on. Others go further and give an estimated mileage that the remaining fuel would allow. Further technology starts to suggest to you where suitable petrol stations may be located.

If we use the oxygen cylinder in equipment failure example, the day when we are not only relying on a gauge will be a big step forward. If the cylinder could estimate how long a journey in the back of an ambulance could be for a certain patient before I would need to change the cylinder, this would be useful, especially if it could warn me in anticipation of that moment when I might need to change. Of course, we can do these calculations manually but as we have already established, to err is human and every backup system might make our patients just that bit safer and eliminate another hole from our cheese.

So when considering how we act on information, we need to be aware of the quality of the information on which we are basing our decision-making. We need to understand, at least in part, how that data is generated and how inaccuracies may occur. Most importantly, we need to start with the clinical information from the patient and not just treat the monitor.

Post-procedures checks

At the end of an episode of using a piece of equipment, how often do you check that it is working adequately before you put it away? Are you sure you clean it before it goes back in the cupboard? Is that 'someone' else's job and if so, whose? What systems do you have in place to report a fault? Who does deal with them? Or is it rather random whether faults get picked up? What could you put in place to change that?

If we now consider more specific examples, I realize that not all of these will be relevant to everyone. However, if you do have a non-clinical role it is still useful to have an understanding of what your clinical colleagues may face.

Drug errors

Drugs—prescribing errors

We often joke about the handwriting of doctors. I have used the retort in the past that 'it took me years of training to write that badly!'. But joking aside, when we are prescribing is not the time to have illegible handwriting that could in any way be ambiguous. It needs to be printed in capitals without the use of abbreviations. There seems to be disagreement or almost cyclical changes over my prescribing history whether we want it written tds (*ter die sumendus*) or 8° to represent a drug to be given every 8 hours or three times a day.

It is possible to prescribe the wrong drug, the wrong dose, or the wrong frequency, or a mixture of those three.

It is also possible to have prescribed drugs that may have interactions between them. It is possible to have the drug prescribed more than once. This is more likely if there are multiple charts or multiple sections of the same chart.

An omission from a chart can be just as dangerous.

The ambiguity from a poor prescription can occur during the dispensing process, the preparation process, or the administering of the drug.

Preparation

We will start by considering drugs that we can inject. When considering the simplest end of the spectrum, we may simply draw up a neat drug from a container of some description (often an ampoule) into a syringe with a drawing up needle. So where might the errors occur?

Imagine now the stress of a patient who has suddenly deteriorated and the staff member rushes to the cupboard. There is no clear system to the way the drug packets are stored. It is supposed to be by alphabetical order but is that by the generic name of the drug or the actual name or the preparation? The colours of the boxes are not standardized and if you change manufacturer the drug box looks different. They take the box off the shelf and read the name out loud. Having located the correct box, are the right drugs in that box? Or is it possible that someone didn't use some ampoules yesterday and tried to save money and put them away but into the wrong box. The patient is dying. This treatment is the one that might save them. The time pressure is on. We need to locate the appropriate size syringe and remove it from its wrapper. We must find a drawing up needle and put it on the end of the syringe (having again removed its sterile wrapper). We should label the syringe with a prepared label if possible to save time. We insert the needle tip into the ampoule and invert both the ampoule and the syringe. Whilst we pull on the plunger of the syringe we read aloud the drug name and dose and strength if appropriate. We verbalize the expiry date and check that the solution is not cloudy. We should also say aloud the dose that we want to give and how many millilitres of liquid that would be. And still the pressure of the patient's life being saved by the contents of the syringe is upon us. Melodramatic? Perhaps, but a not infrequent occurrence in acute areas. In that setting, I wonder how many of those checks may just not quite happen as they are intended to happen.

If we make things a little more complicated and now we have to calculate how many milligrams of a drug we need (let's call it drug A) (which involves a calculation and then only drawing up part of an ampoule) and then we need to dilute it up (perhaps with some salty water called saline) to make it into a different strength. Now the process is more complicated there is a higher cognitive workload and there are more potential layers of cheese. The errors can occur in the calculation of the amount of drug A, in the drawing up of drug A, in the calculation of the amount of the diluent required, or in the drawing up of the diluent.

If you are one of those involved in this type of preparation phase, how do you reduce your chances of making an error?

I think it is important not to underestimate how important it is that you are not interrupted during this process. It can be useful to have a 'safe place' for preparation which could be behind closed doors or in an area that is marked off, perhaps with a line painted on the floor. Everyone knows that when someone is in that area they are not to be interrupted unless it is life threatening.

The process needs to be standardized. Unfortunately there is, as yet, not sufficient research to identify the safest practice. The key thing is getting into a routine of breaking the process down into steps and giving each the attention it deserves.

Of course, there are other ways of preparing drugs which include preparation in a pharmacy or specialized environment and each of these brings with it its own ways that errors may occur. Be error aware.

Identification errors

It sounds simple to have the right prescription/drug chart for the right patient and to give them the right drug at the right time by the right route. However, it is not. Every possible combination of this error has occurred.

We can pick up the wrong chart or take a drug to the wrong patient or take the wrong drug to the right patient or we can take the right drug to the right patient but give it by the wrong route. The wrong drug also covers giving a patient something to which we know they are allergic.

What safety checks do you have in place to try and prevent this? How could you improve the process to make it even safer? This is sometimes called 'active identification'.

We need to think about whether we should be doing this on our own or checking it with another person. If we are checking it with someone else I request that we start to consider more closely how we go about that (see Example 5.7).

Example 5.7 Checking of drugs with someone else

Imagine that I have called you over on a busy ward to come and check something with me. You have many other tasks on your mind. I show you a chart, read out the name for you, and tell you how I have already interpreted the prescription. I show you the drug that I have prepared and read the label on the side of the bottle and the expiry date out loud to you. I have only expected you to mutter yes, at various points along the process. I sign in the box and ask you to countersign underneath. Safe?

Er, no! If I ask closed questions or say something along the lines of, 'this is x isn't it?' you are highly likely to agree with me. If, however, I have already done my checklist and now I ask you to come over and check for me, consider the differences in this approach:

'Please can you check some drugs for my patient, Mrs Rose in bed 5? She is not allergic to anything and is requesting some pain killers for a headache.' When you come over you pick up the drug chart and read aloud, 'this is the drug chart for Mrs Vera Rose, I note from my handover sheet that she is in bed 5 (this is cross checking the information that we are given with another source). I confirm that the chart says that she has no allergies. She last had paracetamol at 10pm last night which is over 8 hours ago. There is no other prescription for that drug on the chart. This is a box of paracetamol 500mg per tablet and the expiry date on the box is May next year. The prescription is for 1 gram, which is two tablets, to be given orally. I assume she is able to take it orally?'. Both of us then attend the patient, check the identity band against the drug chart and confirm verbally with the patient. Again this should be an open question, 'can you confirm your name for me?' not a leading question like, 'Mrs Brown?'. The latter has been a source of many an error. 'And your date of birth?' this is active identification as there are two open questions.

I ask only for you to consider your current practice, my intention is not to be prescriptive in this method. I think more research is required prior to us adopting a standardized approach.

Administration

The next thing to consider is who is doing the administering—the patient, the nurse, the doctor, the relative, or another carer.

If the patient is self-administering there is a whole multitude of different ways we could have an error before we get anywhere near the administration phase. From the time when the GP takes a history and the patient forgets that they are allergic to something, to the electronic typing of the prescription or a problem with the printer, or a failure to sign the prescription. The patient may put the prescription in their bag and forget all about it. There may be a pharmacy error—wrong drug, wrong strength, wrong dose, wrong person, wrong frequency, or simply poor instructions. The patient may misunderstand what they have been told, or be confused, or forget or leave the drugs somewhere. Should all of those steps been successful the patient and the drugs may both arrive home. There are the added problems of being on other drugs, incompatibilities with food stuffs, taking it at the right time and with the right frequency, and not mixing it up with another drug that looks very similar. If we then consider the added complications if it is not in tablet form but involves learning to give yourself an injection, for example, for insulin, a number of times a day. It is a real wonder that drug errors are not more common at home, or is it? Who will be affected by this type of drug error? Who, therefore, might be very focused on getting it right?

If we imagine we are now in a ward setting. A nurse wishes to administer a drug.

If we start with the simple process of giving someone a tablet, how can that go wrong? Assuming we have no prescribing error or identity errors, what else could happen?

Assuming that most oral drugs are kept in packets in blister packs, this is where the next errors in the chain may occur. If someone has previously taken out the strip of tablets and then returned them to the wrong box, it is now possible to pick up the correct box and take out the wrong drug. The boxes may look the same but contain different drugs. There is currently no system for control of the appearance of drug packets—I think there should be. The drugs may have very similar names. There may be two packets with the same drug but at different strengths (e.g. a 25mg tablet and a 50mg tablet). Throw into the mix a busy ward with high noise levels and regular interruptions and it starts to become quite easy to visualize why drug errors are commonplace.

We need to change some of our systems. We need to introduce some simple safety technologies to enhance this process. We also need to be more disciplined in never interrupting someone who is doing a drug round or drawing up drugs.

Problems with the administration of drugs in syringes are even easier to envisage. A drug that was intended to go into a vein could be given into a muscle. A drug that was intended for an epidural could be given into a vein. The drip that used to be in the vein could have moved and now be under the skin and so the drug ends up under the skin too. There may be more than one drug set to run into a vein but the drugs are not compatible, when they mix they form a precipitate. There may be a drip line full of air that isn't seen when the syringe in a pump is changed. There may be lots of syringes all in a row in pumps and they are mixed up and the dose changed on the wrong one. The pump may fail. The doctor may simply pick up the wrong syringe from the several that are in the tray and give the wrong drug. The drug may have been labelled incorrectly so that even when the clinician checks the syringe has the correct name on it, it is still the wrong drug. There may have been maintenance people working on the pipeline gases and somehow they have reattached them incorrectly so the oxygen and nitrous oxide are now coming out of the wrong hoses.

I have seen/been in a department when every single one of these errors has occurred in my career.

Parallel types of errors can occur with medical gases. The gases can be given to the wrong patient, at the wrong time, at the wrong dose, it can be the wrong gas or the wrong delivery method can be used.

Timing

A delay in administration of some drugs can be critical, for example, antibiotics in neutropenic sepsis. The delay can be due to failure to see the patient soon enough, failure to make the diagnosis, failure to know the treatment, failure to look up a guideline, failure to follow the protocol, failure to prescribe the drug, writing it illegibly, failing to tell someone you have prescribed the drug, failure for someone to give the drug, and so on. There are a list of treatments that are time critical, for example, in heart attacks and strokes.

The frequency of a drug may also be vital. If it is given too frequently it can result in overdose, if it is given too infrequently then the treatment may not be effective. As with the wrong frequency, the wrong dose can result in either too much drug or too little drug and either option can have serious complications.

Wrong route

I have already talked earlier in the book about the multiple cases of vincristine being given via the wrong route. I have talked also about how there is now a new system being developed where an intravenous syringe will no longer attach to a spinal needle. This will help to reduce this error. I would of course love to say, eliminate this error but no matter how safe you think you have made a system, a cheese hole that you have not yet thought of can happen. For example, in this case if you somehow ended up with the wrong drug in the wrong syringe at the pharmacy end, you could still attach the spinal syringe to the spinal needle with an interlocking mechanism and it could still be an error.

My intention is not that you should be paranoid, but it is that you should be error aware. 'Where is the next error going to happen?' is a healthy mind set from a safety perspective.

Wrong equipment/wrong technique

We have already alluded to the fact that the drug can be prepared in a syringe and then given via the wrong route. It may also be that the wrong needle is attached for a particular purpose (too big if it was intended to be just under the skin or too small if the intention is it should be reaching as far as the muscle).

Drip sets are another source of errors if the wrong type of drip set is used for the wrong fluid or the wrong patient group. This links in also with the administration of blood products when the giving set may also be relevant.

Human tissue, blood products, and transplantation

The first step in the process is the collection. There are a variety of processes, preparation, and storage that are then required and this may then be followed by cross-matching.

The error may occur during the administration phase in a similar way to giving a drug. It might be the wrong patient, it could be the wrong blood/product/organ, it could be given via the wrong route or at the wrong time. There may be a delay in getting the product or it may be given too quickly or too slowly. The wrong amount might be given (too little or too much).

There may be a problem with the instruments or sterility used at any phase of the process from collection to delivery. There can be incompatibilities between blood products and some drugs.

Instruments

The sterility of instruments can be an issue but is usually discovered before they are used. What is far worse is the instrument that is left in the patient during a surgical procedure. Despite rigorous checking procedures that should now be in place, this event is still occurring. We have to ask ourselves why? How is the checklist performed? Does it engage both of the checkers? Are people trying to multi- task at this phase of the procedure when it is nearly the end? Are they interrupted or distracted or under time pressure? How could we make it safer?

Another issue with instruments can occur when one set of equipment is not compatible with another. For example, a light source with a different laparoscope that won't fit together but the patient is already asleep when it is discovered.

Beds

I admit that it sounds rather strange to think of errors and problems to do with beds!

My first bug bear is a particular bed design that obviously never considered that a patient might need emergency treatment whilst in it. It is possible to remove the head of the bed but there is then a large solid metal bar at shin level at the head end that keeps all clinical staff about twelve inches away from the bed. If there is an emergency and you need to reach the head of the patient you must develop the arms of Mr Tickle (a reference to a book from my childhood).

There have been errors associated with mechanical and electrical bed failures and problems with the hardness of mattresses when trying to deliver lifesaving treatment such as CPR (cardiopulmonary resuscitation). There have also been problems with people trapped in bed rails or have fallen because of a lack of them.

Key points from Chapters 1–5

- We all make mistakes. We can get better at anticipating them with practice. Are you looking at how to avoid your next one?

- We need to embed an open culture.

- There should be an inquisitive approach to error that seeks out the learning and shares it: the learning culture.

- The new error checklist—the SHEEP sheet—helps gather more information following an actual event or a nearly event. The SHEEP sheet can be used for trend analysis.

◆ Information flow across an organization can be achieved using a brief/debrief model using Debbie's Diamond.

◆ Systems errors are commonly part of the holes in the Swiss cheese model and should feature in the solutions for improved safety.

◆ Things are not always what they seem: avoid assumption.

◆ 'What am I missing here?' is a healthy question to keep asking.

◆ If the hierarchy is too steep, the team will not feel able to challenge the leader when they are making a mistake. We all make mistakes.

◆ If there is a flat hierarchy, no natural leader emerges, ask the question, 'Who's leading?'.

◆ Followership is a much overlooked and important skill to have. This can involve being assertive enough to speak up if things are about to go wrong.

◆ We will all push someone else's buttons. We can't change the other person, only ourselves.

◆ We need to become more aware of how we are impacting on others (increase our self-awareness). This might begin with knowing our preferred learning style, team role, and our personality type (MBTI).

◆ Once we know who we are more likely to 'clash' with, we can try and blend in a bit better (self-management) to avoid conflict.

◆ If we do end up in conflict we will behave in an assertive way (this is completely different from aggressive although the terms are often misused) and aim to find a win–win situation.

◆ A good leader will be able to switch to using four different leaderships styles when appropriate and will avoid micro-management or pacesetting. (This pacesetting style currently dominates the NHS in both clinical and non-clinical leaders.)

◆ Remember when giving feedback and praise:

　◆ Situation Behaviour Impact Change or Continue.

◆ Knowing where everything is and having it laid out in a logical, clearly marked way not only makes it more efficient but it makes it safer.

◆ Standardizing the layout of clinical areas decreases errors.

◆ If you are doing a transfer, plan and plan some more.

- Try not to interrupt others. If you are interrupted yourself, start the task again if you can and watch for errors.

- Try not to stand over patients in their beds and talk down to them. Always imagine how they might be feeling.

- SBAR—situation, background, assessment, recommendation/request— is good for handovers of information, especially on the phone.

- 'Active identification' needs to become standard practice with all drug administration and before any procedure and before any clinical interaction.

- It is possible to design equipment to eliminate layers of cheese and to decrease the chance of error.

- Being adequately trained on a piece of equipment is essential. Subsequent skill maintenance is also essential, particularly if the kit is used infrequently.

- Training with simulation offers an alternative for acquiring and maintaining skills.

6

The 'P' of SHEEP: Personal

It doesn't involve expertise; all you need is a mind which is good at guessing, some courage, and a natural talent for interacting with people

Plato (429–347 BC)

Gorgias, Section 463b (translated by Robin Waterfield). Reproduced from Elizabeth Knowles, Oxford Dictionary of Quotations, Seventh Edition, Oxford, UK, Copyright © 2009, by permission of Oxford University Press

Introduction

It is time to consider the 'P' of the algorithm (see Figure 6.1). I want to focus on our staff themselves and think about how their lives can impact on their work. This is where self-awareness and then self-management really begin.

We will start with some of the easier topics that are more tangible.

Physiology/pathology

This means how your body works normally and when there is a health problem.

There are basic needs that everyone has: food, water, sleep, and to empty your bowels and urinate. You do not need me to tell you that if any of your basic needs are not met, then you will begin to function less effectively and you are more likely to make a mistake. The interesting thing for me is not that people don't know this, they do know, but that we ask it of each other and of ourselves to compromise these basic functions.

As I ate my sandwich while typing up some research and having a conversation about it at 2.30 pm today, the irony was not wasted on me. Why was it that I had organized my day in such a way that my lunch was not a high priority? Why has

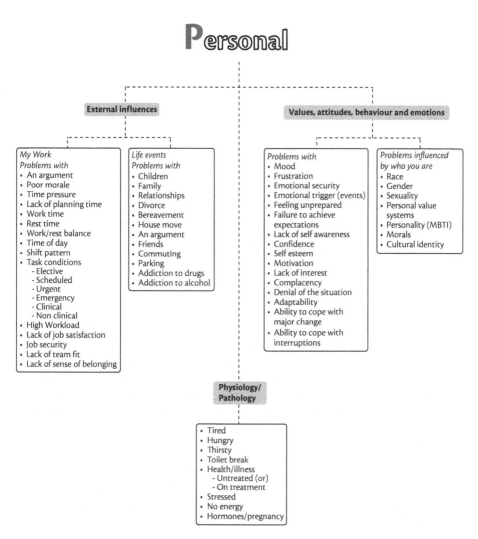

Figure 6.1 'P'—the SHEEP model.

it taken me until I'm writing about it in a book to put it in my diary to remind me to stop for lunch?

I understand this is becoming such a common corporate phenomenon that it is now referred to dining 'al desco'.

I teach the topic regularly, we talk about how concentration levels are lower without adequate gaps or rest breaks and food and water. It is also more difficult to focus if your bladder is distracting you!

Is it that we are simply distracted by the long list of complex tasks that just take over? Is it just bad planning? Is it a sense of martyrdom? Is it that we are 'so' important that nothing will happen without us there? Which of those best fits your setting and what might you do about it?

Fatigue

The tiredness is more serious. There is clear evidence that sleep deprivation impairs performance significantly.

There may be reasons for sleep disturbance at home: small children, snoring partner, health issues (reflux, cough, pain, prostate problem), noisy neighbours, uncomfortable bed, traffic, the weather, the temperature, stressful life event, and many more. My question is, if this is the case, how are going to try and keep these things at manageable levels? Who is in your support network? What might you need to change? Who might you need to see?

If you are one of those who, like me, comes up with good ideas when you are asleep then my tip would be to have paper and a pen by the side of your bed. Capture your idea on the paper and then you can let go of it and go back to sleep more quickly. 'They' say (although I'm not sure who 'they' are) that you should write everything down that might be bothering you or on your mind before you even go to sleep. For me, it is not something that is knowingly bothering me that crops up, it is a new and creative idea and I'm worried that if I don't write it down I will have forgotten it by the morning. If this is relevant to you, I find that scribbling my idea quickly allows me to let go and return to my slumber more quickly.

The other issues related to fatigue in the health setting are those related to the work itself. The patterns of work, the length of the shifts, the rotas, the antisocial hours, and also the nature of the work itself can interfere with our usual diurnal or circadian rhythms as well as reduce the hours available for sleep.

There is evidence that more errors occur on night shifts.

Whilst the hypothesis could be that there are fewer staff on shift at night and, therefore, more errors occur, the evidence points to the fact that we do not have the same level of cognitive ability at night.

Is this due to poorer sleep quality if we are trying to sleep in the day? (Are you interrupted by noisy neighbours who are unaware that you are working nights, for example? Or perhaps you are woken by the phone when one of those lovely automatic dialling services tries to talk to you about insurance?)

Could it be that when we are working nights that we try to do too much and don't actually go to bed for long enough? (You desperately need to go to the bank but it is only open when you should be sleeping and while you are in town you 'just' run a couple of other errands. When you get back, the light is streaming through the window and it is difficult to get off to sleep. All too soon it is time to go to work again!)

Sleep deprivation has been shown to cause the same level of cognitive impairment as alcohol consumption. The majority of people know not to drive and not to operate heavy machinery whilst under the influence of alcohol. I assume also that you would not try to look after a patient nor perform a procedure after you have been drinking, so that begs the question, why is it acceptable when you are tired?

How can we make it safer?

My personal preference when my children were small and I had been up half the night was to be honest. There is a difference between being the mood hoover and leading a 'whinge fest' or to merely state facts. I used to say something along the lines of, 'I haven't had enough sleep so I am more likely to make a mistake today. Please keep an extra check on what I'm doing and if you see me doing anything you are not sure about, please tell me'. The language would vary slightly depending on how well I knew my ODA/ODP/anaesthetic nurse whom I was working alongside. This serves the purpose of introducing an extra check, admitting vulnerability which alters the steepness of the hierarchy, raises error awareness, and makes it OK to challenge me if I am making a mistake. In addition, I would slow down slightly. I would make sure I was using conscious thought rather than automatic. I would double check any calculations I made or prescriptions that I wrote. I also hope that in some tiny way I was role modelling safety-positive behaviour.

On a very sad note there have been some road traffic accidents when people who have worked long shifts have been driving home, some of which have been fatal. I ask that you also drive very carefully when you are tired or consider whether you could sleep first. I also ask you to make sure that the shift lengths of our staff are reasonable. I ask that there are systems in place so people are given some rest breaks. I ask that we in the 'caring' profession start to look after ourselves and each other, in addition to our patients.

If you are someone who struggles to get enough sleep, I include a few tips here. If you go to sleep at the drop of a hat then skip forward to 'toilet breaks'.

Establishing a routine for the half an hour before bedtime is useful. During that time you should stop doing anything that is stimulating your brain, think of it as a pre-sleep time. Your brain needs a bit of wind down time to change modes between two different states. Activities that are thought to have a negative effect in this pre-sleep time include computers, other electronic devices, reading a book, alcohol, drugs, watching television, and anything else that involves you thinking or engaging your brain. Things that might be useful during this time are relaxing activities; think about what that means for you. A warm bath, gentle music (choose it carefully, not stimulating), lower lighting levels, and a good old warm, milky drink. An adequate amount of fresh air and exercise in the preceding day may also be useful. You need to think of it as a 'Pavlov dog'-type moment. You need to do the same thing every night. Only when you have done that 90 times does it count as having established a routine. Take a moment to design yours now.

What will your routine be like? Do you prefer to visualize it or write it down? If you are writing it will it be in pictures or words? Black and white or colour? Paper or computer?

Remember you are designing a routine that will take half an hour and will be the same as many nights a week as possible. I realize you might socialize some nights!

Remember that it takes 90 repeats before you can start to call it a routine. How are you going to make sure you keep on doing it?

I worked with someone who in the same breath told me that they always read a book before they go to sleep and they have dreadful trouble getting to sleep. This was fairly easy to solve.

I would recommend thinking of bed as a place to sleep but there should be no books, television, or electronic devices (laptops, tablets, phones, etc.) in bed. Think about the temperature and the lighting level, and then empty your bladder as you get ready for bed. Think about what you are wearing or not wearing! You need to be comfortable and the temperature of your environment is important. Think also about the pillows—shape, fullness, and number. Consider the covers in terms of how they feel against your skin and the temperature. Once you are in bed consider using a relaxation technique if you think you are still tense. I have included one here if you need it (see Example 6.1).

Example 6.1 Relaxation technique

Turn off the lights and anything else that might distract you. Lie on your back. Adjust your pillows so that you are comfortable. Consider using a small rolled towel under your knees if you need to alleviate any pressure on your lower back. Lie there and shut your eyes. For the first couple of minutes I would like you to ponder on your awareness of the bed. Which bits of you are in contact with the bed? Can you feel the covers on your skin? What is the temperature of the sheets, and the bedcovers, and the air? I want you to pay attention to your breathing. Feel the breath go and out.

As you lie there, thoughts may enter your head. Don't be cross with those thoughts. Ponder why it is that topic that is interesting you right now and then let the thought drift off again.

After a few minutes I want you to focus on your feet. Be aware of your feet. What position are they in? What are they touching? I want you to screw them up tight and hold it for 5 seconds and then release. As you release them, let them become fully relaxed and let them sink deeper into the bed. Take a slow deep breath.

Now I want you to focus on your legs and your buttocks. Be aware of your legs and your buttocks. What position are they in? What are they touching? I want you to tense up your whole legs and buttocks as tight as you can and hold it for 5 seconds and then release. As you release them, let them become fully relaxed and let them sink deeper into the bed. Take a slow deep breath.

Now I want you to focus on your belly and your pelvic floor. I want you to pull in your belly and pull up your pelvic floor. Hold it for 5 seconds and then release. Take a slow deep breath.

I want you to focus on your hands. Be aware of your fingers. What position are they in? What are they touching? I want you to screw them up tight and hold it for 5 seconds and then release. As you release them, let them become fully relaxed and let them sink deeper into the bed. Take a slow deep breath.

Now I want you to focus on your arms and your shoulders. Be aware of your arms and your shoulders. What position are they in? What are they touching? I want you to tense up your whole hands and arms and shoulders as tight as you can and hold it for 5 seconds and then release. As you release them, let them become fully relaxed and let them sink deeper into the bed. Take a slow deep breath.

I want you to take ten slow, conscious breaths focusing on the breath coming in, your chest expanding, and then letting the breath out slowly in a controlled way as you slowly allow your chest to fall.

Take a moment and then roll into your sleeping position and just let go.

One of the commonest misconceptions is that going to sleep is an active process, 'I cannot get to sleep'. This begs the question where is sleep and how do we find it?

I think of it completely differently. Sleep is a natural state when we recharge our batteries. It is a time when we go into 'standby' mode and as such we need to 'power down'. By allowing your brain and body to relax, it allows the waves of sleep to arrive in your brain and let them take over the control of the brain's rhythm instead.

As a junior doctor, working many more hours than would now be allowed, I perfected the art of the catnap or power nap. I could sleep anywhere, in any position. I could recharge my batteries in 50 minutes if I had to. I have found this is less effective as I've got older!

For almost 20 years I put people to sleep for a living. Of course, this is a drug-induced sleep and is completely different from natural sleep. This is something that we don't seem to have grasped culturally. There is another commonly held misconception that by taking a pill/prescribing a pill we can sort out sleep. I completely disagree. The quality of restorative sleep from a drug-induced sleep is not comparable. Drug-induced sleep does not result in the same phases of sleep and not the same types of changes in the electricity of the brain waves if you measure them. The majority will result in a slightly altered perception and cognitive function and 'sluggishness' when you do wake up. It would be an enormous step forward if we stopped prescribing sleeping tablets and started tackling the problem with a long-term solution in mind rather than a quick fix. Yes true, it probably is developing into a soapbox moment without me having pre-framed it! If we stopped prescribing these drugs (I mean to start by not starting anyone new on them), we would stop a huge number of addictions from starting. We would save a lot of money that we could spend on employing psychologists/counsellors to help teach relaxation and deal with the underlying problems! Of course, I am not naïve enough to believe it is simple if they are already addicted.

The toilet break

Having worked predominantly in the NHS for 20 years, I have no way of know-ing if it is a phenomenon that is unique to our industry. It is unacceptable for me to leave a patient whilst in theatre, unless I am relieved by another anaesthe-tist, whilst they are under anaesthesia.

This means that if you are doing a long case that lasts all day and you are on your own you have to develop a massive bladder capacity! This can also be the case if there is a very busy list with a high turnover. I know this is also a problem in many other areas of the NHS—wards, clinics, and non-clinical areas alike.

I want you to consider how to look after yourself better and to how to look after the other staff around you. I want you to plan little mini breaks which involve a mouthful of food, a drink, and a toilet break. I am not in the realms of what you are legally allowed which is far more than that but I'm thinking about patient safety. I want you to be able to concentrate and to be less likely to make a mistake.

Staff health/illness

I have seen an intriguing array of approaches to staff illness over my career. Attitudes seem to range from the stoical, Blitz-esk 'Carry On' to the one sneeze and it is 'flu'. There are organizational systems and cultural issues at play here.

There are organizations that favour the stick approach. If you are off sick, even for a day or so, this results in a return to work interview. If you are off three times in a certain time frame, there are certain procedures to be followed as the process escalates. Within these systems I have observed differences between the professional groups. Some of the doctors reading this will have no concept of the return to work interview or at least no personal experience of it. Those of you in other professional groups will be all too familiar with the sentiments I'm expressing. Why is it that there are differences? Which groups are getting it right? How can we reduce the double standards within the system? Do you believe in a carrot or a stick?

My personal thoughts are that working in healthcare is unique. We deal with sick patients. We don't have some sort of 'super' immunity just because we have entered the caring profession. It is logical that we have increased illness exposure and that we are at risk of 'catching things'. To punish people for being ill is inhumane and does nothing to look after our staff. I think it should stop. If you make people come to work when they ill they are not only more likely to infect others, potentially including our patients, but they are also more likely to make a mistake. I shall just say that bit again, they are more likely to make a mistake, and so why is it a good idea for them to be there?

Yes, of course, there is a subset of people who swing the lead. I understand that there needs to be a system to explore this behaviour but it does not mean that all of our staff should be made to suffer, nor patient safety be compromised.

I am, of course, aware of the behaviour associated with healthcare professionals (especially medical students and I can say that because once upon a time I was one) who can list 20 causes of a headache at the drop of a hat. Whilst brain tumour may be on the list of differentials, it is far more likely in this case to be post-alcohol consumption recovery phase or a good old-fashioned hangover (or it was when I was a medical student!). We will return to the topic of alcohol later. Whilst being a bit of a hypochondriac is a problem with some, there are others who believe it is a sign of weakness to ever take time off and are at risk of running themselves into an early grave. We should be aiming at a happy medium. Like anyone else we should seek medical advice appropriately and not try and manage it ourselves (which evidence shows we do poorly). Whilst you can self-certify for a week in most places, you should see your GP or occupational health and not simply try to carry out the old adage, 'physician, heal thyself'.

If it is a chronic (long-term) condition, there should be a clear plan of how this will be managed and patient care must come into these conversations, no matter how difficult that may be. There are healthcare professionals who lose their sight, who develop a tremor, who have cancer, who have neuromuscular diseases, mental health issues, and addiction, and so on, just the same spectrum as our patients. We need to be honest with ourselves for the benefit of our patients if we are no longer up to the job.

We have a fantastic network of occupational health physicians, nurses, and their teams: please use them and seek their advice and support.

Stress

Stress. It is a funny word that means different things to different people. When I was a student I was taught about a series of reactions that caused the release of certain 'chemicals' into the bloodstream, which nerves were involved, and which organs. I was taught how we can measure changes and when this 'stress response' might be induced. But that is not the approach I wish to consider today. I wish to consider a much more personal, colloquial version. There is a long-term stress during a life event (we will give these a whole section later) or something far quicker after what I am going to call a 'trigger'.

What does stress mean to you? How do you know it is starting? What are the very first signs of it in you? Where does it start? Is it the same response for different triggers?

The next time it happens, pay attention to those feelings. Was there anything that happened even earlier to tell you it was coming?

What are your triggers? Or put another way, what pushes your buttons?

Take a moment to write a list or at least construct one in your head before you read my personal examples. How many have you got?

Mine include a whole myriad of things, some of which are actual triggers and some of which just alter my threshold for a trigger. I am more likely to be triggered if I am already tired, under a high cognitive workload, hungry, chocolate or caffeine deprived, late (I hate being late), if someone spontaneously dumps work on me with a short deadline (I am horribly organized and I like to be in control), if it is raining or if I am cold, and there are many more. Of course, there are the big triggers—bereavement, house move, divorce, or major life events. Examples of my simple everyday triggers include laziness, rudeness/lack of manners, slow computers, an argument with someone I love or having to tell off the children, inefficiency, witnessing someone speaking about someone else behind their back, time wasting, red tape, indecision, micro-management, mood hoovers, selfishness, ego (there is no 'me' in team—I hate the phrase but agree with the sentiment), bullying, a blinkered approach, the phrases of the time (currently 'blue sky thinking', 'outside the box', ' . . . with respect . . . ' The last of which means I am about to say something that is completely disrespectful) and standing in a very long queue while the process could be optimized to make it all move much faster, in fact, I'm probably not very good at waiting full stop. I could probably fill a chapter! (I'm not sure if that means I am self-aware or just have a long list of triggers and need to be more tolerant!)

I think it is important to understand yourself. It may be that you have to deal with some of those stresses right before there is a clinical emergency. We need to be able to manage ourselves sufficiently so that we do not let our stresses impact on those around us. How do you do that? Have you ever given it any thought?

When there is a trigger, it may well be out of your hands. The bit that is yours to own is the response you let the trigger invoke in you. You actually have a choice in how you let it impact on you. Are you going to let it rile you?

What coping mechanisms have you mastered? How do you call upon them? What are you like under pressure?

Here are a few ideas that might help with resilience. Feel free to take only those that you fancy as not all tools work for all people. I confess to having what I call a Batman approach: a utility belt with all of my tools tucked in it and I simply reach for the right tool as and when I need it.

The first metaphor that I wish to share isn't mine and I think there are a few versions of it. I want you to imagine a pint glass and that you have filled it with ping pong balls. Is it full? Now I would like you to take some small pebbles (about the same size as a 10-pence piece) and put those into the glass. Now is it full? Following the beach theme, I would like you to fill the glass with sand. The sand now fills the spaces around both the ping pong balls and the pebbles. Now, is it full? Now I want you to take some beer (other beverages are available) and pour it in. The beer fills all of the air spaces that were in the sand. Only now is it truly full.

I want you to think about what is most important to you in your life. What is the really important 'stuff' that if you took it away your life would be unbearable? For me, this is my close family. These are your ping pong balls. Now I want you to think about the things are really important to you but a step down from your absolute highest priority. For me, this is my friends, my house, my job, and enough money. These are your pebbles. We each have our own priorities in life. By the time we are getting to the differences between brands of clothing or colours of paint on a wall, I am beyond my sand level. In times of 'stress' focus on the ping pong balls and try to keep the pebbles going but forget about the rest. I have heard an alternative version of the metaphor which is slightly more tongue in cheek: no matter how full your life may seem, there is always space for a beer between friends.

So, what coping mechanisms do you use effectively? You will have mastered more than you realize. Some of them are useful but caution is necessary as some of them may be detrimental.

I have asked for a few examples that people use. A close friend uses what they call 'sloping shoulders'—they just let it slide straight off so they don't carry it around with them. Another uses the philosophy, 'if I can't change it, why worry about it'. Another unpacks their 'back-pack' before they leave work so they don't take it all home with them. Someone else has a 'too hard pile' where they can leave things on hold until they have the emotional wherewithal to deal with it. I think this one resembles my putting it in a box and holding it at arm's length and only taking the lid off when I am ready and then perhaps only to peek and put the lid back on. Eventually I unpack the box in manageable, bite-size chunks (apologies for the mixed metaphors!). There is also the famous idea of 'how do we eat an elephant?'—one bite at a time.

In an acute (sudden, emergency) setting, I think the two-breath technique is very helpful. As far as I'm aware this one is used by NASA but it is used in other settings too. It is sometimes called a 'hold' or a 'time out' or a 'five-second count' or sometimes 'ten seconds'. No matter what you call it, the ideas are the same. Once you identify where your stress response starts (and the earlier you learn to identify that the better), you can try this to stop it taking hold of you. Stop what you are doing. Acknowledge the feeling. Take two slow, deep breaths and own the stress response. Now put it to one side and allow yourself to continue with a clear head. After the emergency has happened and it is over you can allow the reality to hit home and then have a really good debrief to look for the learning that can take place.

So what does your stress response feel like? I realize for those of you who would rather think than feel I am potentially asking a challenging question. The answers I usually get are 'heart racing', butterflies in the stomach or the chest, flushing red in either the neck or the face or both, sweaty palms, generalized agitation, wringing of hands, biting of nails, or being able to hear your pulse. You need to learn to identify your own response.

Does that sound too 'fluffy bunny' for you? To answer the cynics I will say this. Anaesthetics is sometimes described as '90% boredom and 10% oh s . . t!!' As such, over the last almost 20 years I have faced a lot of emergencies, a large number of which were life threatening, which needed a cool head and needed to be resolved in a short amount of time. I have found the two-breath technique very useful. It might be worth a go if you don't already have a coping mechanism for that type of sudden stressor. I used it way before I heard that NASA used it! I find it useful before I give a big talk. I find it useful when I feel on the verge of shouting at my children. I have taught it to people on my courses and they have also found it useful.

Why does it work? I have two answers for that. I will give you the woollier answer first (no, that wasn't an attempt at a sheep joke!). If you are interested in learning more about self-awareness, I would recommend that you explore the concepts of mindfulness. There are books and courses and indeed a whole movement that helps you explore this more fully. It helps you be more aware of living in the present. I realize this will be a step too far for some but for those of you with an open mind, I recommend that it is a concept worth exploring.

There is also an answer that will suit those of you who seek a more measurable scientific response. I was at a conference and Pam Kato asked for a volunteer. As I am not exactly known for being 'quiet and retiring', I stepped forward and joined her on the stage. She has developed a computer game that is linked via a series of sensors on your fingers to some derived variables linked to your stress response. In effect, it is possible to 'visualize' how stressed you are or perhaps how in control you are of how stressed you are. It gives you feedback if you can control your 'nerves' as there is no joystick or buttons to control the game—only how you are feeling. I was told that despite the fact that I was sitting on a stage at a conference with everyone watching me, I was too calm! When she enquired about my job, there seemed to be an acknowledgement that that explained it! The game was in its early stages at that time and has since been released.

So, the good news is it is a skill and like other skills it can be learnt and honed with practice. I would of course far rather we practised in a simulated environment rather than waiting for the real stresses of real emergencies to overwhelm us.

In dealing with stress, I want you to consider your work–life balance. It is important that you have one! How is it that you relax? When you come home do you prefer to recharge your batteries with company or on your own? Do you prefer a hobby or activity, or prefer to sit and do nothing in front of the television, or lie in a candlelit bath with music playing? Find whatever way suits you, but do it often enough. In our line of work, you need some 'down time' or 'me time'. Think for a moment about what you would like. How are you going to make sure you build it into your routine?

Michael West points out that a number of factors have been shown to make us happier: love, exercise, green spaces, and caring for other people were amongst the factors that made a difference. How are you going to bring those into your life too?

Our patients and their relatives will often find their 'healthcare episode' stressful. It can be a strange place, filled with unfamiliar faces and machines, and even with its own language, and there are huge emotional undertones relating to illness and mortality. We should also know how to acknowledge these stress responses in our patients and help them to learn to cope.

Why am I bothering to focus on stress? Yerkes and Dodson found that stress or very high levels of 'arousal' adversely affect performance. Those that can cope better with stress are considered to be more resilient. Learning this adaptive response to challenge builds our survival mechanisms. If you are less resilient stress can wear you down and have a negative impact on you.

Hormones/pregnancy/no energy

I admit it is a rather sweeping heading. There are many reasons why we might report to have 'no energy'. Some of those would be things to which we have already alluded—missing the basics: inadequate food, drink, sleep, and rest. A lack of energy may be physiological, psychological, or pathological: it can be due to illness or hormonal imbalance or part of a normal physiological process. For me, the absolute classic was early pregnancy. I remember being so tired after a day's work that when I arrived through the door I would lie on the floor as even climbing the stairs seemed insurmountable at that moment. I have since confirmed I am not alone with this experience. Whilst some breeze through pregnancy, for others it is debilitating. I had a colleague who was sick every day for the entire 40 weeks of her pregnancy. It was incredibly challenging for her to give anaesthetics when she had to run out regularly to be sick. I was luckier in that I suffered hideous nausea but no actual vomiting. I have found that those women who have had an easy pregnancy can be judgemental, let alone some of the reactions of male colleagues. These attitudes are completely unacceptable and must not go unchallenged.

I think we need to set up better support networks for our pregnant staff. It is useful if you talk to someone who has already managed to juggle pregnancy and work (and later on children and work) and remain sane. If it is not hormonal/pregnancy/illness and you still feel that you have no energy, then this bit is for you. I want you to have a really big, honest think for a moment. Are you eating well? You don't need me to tell you what that means, but I would like you to think about timing as well as quality. What about drinking enough water and limiting alcohol to a safe level? The next thing to consider is sleep. Do you manage to get enough sleep of a good quality?

Problems due to issues outside the work environment

Children

If we start to consider some of the pressures that go hand in hand with having children we could consider them as physical, emotional and psychological, financial and practical. It can be physically demanding to be woken at night every night over a long time frame. It can be psychologically demanding sharing milestones, illnesses, successes, and failures as they take the journey from dependent baby, through toddler, primary school to the teenage years, and the readiness to leave the coop. Then the life cycles begin all over again but with the different perspective of being a grandparent. There are the financial pressures of feeding and clothing and housing extra mouths. There are the practical pressures of school runs and holiday time with no school and the joy of an unexpected inset day. The emotional roller coasters of living with 'Kevin and Perry' can result in a stressful home life (if that makes no sense to you, try 'YouTube'. It was a television comedy about teenagers which demonstrates a clever observational study of behaviour and uses it for fun).

It is unsurprising, therefore, that some of those pressures will impact on us at work. I have always found the journey to and from work to be a useful time to change from mummy mode to work mode or vice versa. For those of you who are old enough, there used to be a children's programme when I was growing up with a scarecrow that could change his head for different situations. I think I have to achieve something parallel.

A work–life balance can be difficult to achieve. It is incredibly common for people (I think there are gender differences) to worry about how to do both roles to the best of their ability. There are compromises when juggling so many variables and it is possible to feel that either work or home life is suffering or indeed both. I hope if you fall in this category you will take comfort from how very normal those feelings are.

However negative that may have sounded, I love my children enormously and let us never forget the joy and happiness that they can bring too.

Family

Children are only one of many types of family commitment. It may be that we have ageing relatives or other people dependant on us for help and support. Very parallel situations can occur to those already mentioned, but each situation has its own unique combination of challenges. Decisions about whether a parent is safe living alone or watching their health slowly deteriorate or dementia tighten its grasp can be incredibly challenging and can be present over a long time frame.

People refer to a cycle where parents look after children and then later in life the children have to parent the parents. This can be difficult for both sides. It is difficult to adapt to the changed roles. It can be heart-wrenching to watch independent adults become dependent again. Do not underestimate the effect this may have on you.

It is important that you think about yourself within this scenario. Try to build a support network for yourself and make sure that you get some 'down time'. It is much better to share with your line manager or a supportive colleague that you are under these pressures and to plan 'double checks', rather than just soldier on and then make a massive error into the bargain!

Relationships—partners/spouses

I could probably write a whole book on just this tiny subheading (and perhaps one day I will!) but for now let's just stick to a few principles.

We can start by considering casual or short term versus something more long term. I wish to focus on how relationships may influence you at work.

If we start with the short-term option: it may be that it suits some people not to commit to something longer term. This may be something about personality, life stage, life choice, attitude to commitment, opportunities, or other factors. It is up to you to think about how this may impact on your work. Do you have the emotional wherewithal to cope with that lifestyle? Is there any emotional baggage that you are carrying with you? I do ask that if you opt for multiple partners that you do it safely, as this not only impacts on your own health but potentially that of your patients.

Long-term relationships can, of course, have just as many consequences and perhaps more. There is the finding and testing out phase, the honeymoon period where there is romance and excitement, and then a transition phase into something more regular. There may be a decision to cement that 'regular' phase into something more permanent. At any of these phases there may be a break up initiated in a one-sided way or by mutual agreement.

It is easy to see how a break-up phase may have a negative impact on your work. There are a series of reactions that occur that parallel a bereavement reaction: denial, grief, guilt, anger, adjustment, and healing can happen in varying amounts over varying time frames.

Divorce can be very traumatic for the couple themselves, for any children involved, for each of their extended families, and for joint friends who struggle with their loyalties.

My very clear advice if one of your team is going through this is *not* to give them advice but listen instead. We have a tendency in healthcare to assume, because we are in a caring profession, that we have the answers! We also have a tendency to want to want to fix things. I want you to listen. Just listen and not offer your advice. Do not draw parallels to your own life. Listen some more. Do show empathy in your own words but something along the lines of 'that sounds rough' or 'that sounds like a lot to be dealing with'. Do ask questions to help them explore what they are going to do next. Do offer to see if there is anything you can do to help but don't have a solution in your head when you say it. I would thoroughly recommend Relate if a relationship is struggling whether it might be salvageable or not. They are trained to help people through the transitions, rather than from a well-intending healthcare professional.

Do explain to someone at work, even if you don't want everyone to know your business. You/they will undoubtedly be distracted, no matter how hard you/they try. You/they are only human. Paying more attention to tasks associated with risk is important. Slow down and double check things.

Happy relationships

On a happier note: a good relationship has a positive effect on us and a positive effect on our patients. It can give you love, support, listening and offloading, sharing, de-stressing, and much more.

A light-hearted bit of pseudo-science follows: **Debbie's top tips for choosing a partner!** It seems that there are a few traits that might make a difference to finding someone with whom you might be compatible.

It is nothing new to understand that having similar thoughts about finances (thrifty versus extravagant) can save arguments. So an understanding of whether you would rather save it or spend it and an approach to risk can be useful. Similarly, having an idea about whether each of you wants children or not, will be beneficial. Although I recommend that early conversations do not venture near either of those topics! The topic of religion might also be useful at some point, not only which type but almost more importantly 'how much' or with what strength of feeling? All of these are easy if you are using a computer dating agency and you simply tick some boxes but less easy to bring up into a conversation when you have only just met.

Here a few other topics for you both to consider.

◆ Are you a morning person or a night owl?

◆ Do you like to be organized and on time or are you not worried about being late?

◆ Would you like to plan a holiday in advance (maybe weeks or months ahead) or happily not know where you were going off to tomorrow?

◆ Do you like to talk through your day out loud or would you rather recharge your batteries quietly on your own?

◆ Do you like sex every day or once a week or less?

I am not saying that if you uncover big differences in any of these spectrums that it definitely won't work but it will take more work.

I am also a believer in 'those who play together—stay together', so what hobbies might you be able to share? How is it that you are going to build a friendship? How are you going to maintain it?

Communication and compromise are key relationship skills. An understanding of how to be assertive (remember this is not the same as aggressive) is useful so that you can express your feelings honestly and not let a problem fester. For me, key values include trust and mutual respect. You must explore what are important to you.

I am an old-fashioned romantic and I believe in love. I also think that a strong friendship is vital.

Whilst no relationship is perfect, there should be a balance of good outweighing bad. I am not saying we should throw the towel in the moment a relationship starts to impact negatively on us. In fact, I usually advocate that you have to take the rough with the smooth but there should be thresholds for poor behaviour within a relationship beyond which we should not allow things to progress.

A bad relationship can have a very negative impact on your ability to function at work. Some challenging content follows.

Abusive relationships

Those of us in the health service receive an annual update on child protection training and rightly so. I am not going to repeat that here as it is mandated that you should know about it.

We spend rather less time learning about adult domestic abuse and yet it is far more common. This can take the form of emotional, sexual, or physical abuse or a combination of those. It can be from a partner, family member, or friend. I am going to focus on the most common which is from a partner.

It happens in many ways, but here are a few warning signs to look out for. It often begins with subtle changes around control. There can be an element of belittling and undermining of self-confidence. The abused person often expresses a desire to 'keep the peace' or 'wanting to please' so they adopt a more passive role. The abuser gradually over time takes more decisions. There may be controls imposed over the finances or freedom to go out by the abusive partner. The power distance relationship (hierarchy) within the relationship becomes very steep. It often stems from a need to control. There can be threats to this hierarchy that can trigger an increase in control. (For example, a promotion at work of the victim can challenge the steepness of the perceived hierarchy. This can trigger an increase in the undermining behaviour or an escalation of the abuse.) The progression between control and abuse can be incredibly slow so that the victim is almost unaware of when the changes took place. One day there is a further step forward, a temper, but the victim tends to blame themselves for the trigger for the temper or maybe they are blamed for the trigger by the abuser. Whilst there may be an 'it won't happen again' approach, it usually does and it can escalate in force or frequency.

If this is happening to you or you suspect that it is happening to someone you know, only the person themselves can decide when they wish to get help. Once that moment has arrived, the Domestic Abuse Unit of your local police can be incredibly supportive and subtle in its approach. I would also suggest Relate, even if you go on your own and not as a couple.

My top tips if you are faced with a colleague in this setting include some of the following. Do not offer people advice. Do listen. Do not judge, you have no idea about the complexity of the problems they face. Give them time. Treat them as normally as possible; they are still the same person. Let them make their own decisions but ask them if there is anything you could do to help.

If it is you who is going through the abuse consider the contacts I have already mentioned. Whilst at work, invoke the safety-positive behaviour that I mentioned with divorce. Keep your patients safe. I hope you will also feel strong enough to make yourself safe too.

Arguments and conflict

We have discussed conflict in the human interaction chapter but do not underestimate the effect that an argument will have on you. It may mean that you remain distracted afterwards as it plays on your mind. So just to make your day go even more smoothly, you will make an error too! It is a good time to be error aware.

Bereavement

There are a series of emotional reactions that are often associated with bereavement. They can occur in any order and in varying amounts. They include anger, denial, and blame. There can be a sort of acceptance with time but not always. How people adjust to this loss is very variable and depends on multiple factors.

If you are working with someone who is recently bereaved, here are some of my thoughts. Do listen. Don't tell them stories of when someone you knew died; leave it to be about them and their loss. Don't pretend nothing has happened. Empathy is good, 'I was sorry to hear your news'. Silence is OK. Whether or not someone likes to be touched is very personal and it is a huge spectrum; some like to be held while they sob their heart out, others will recoil at the slightest hint of physical contact. Go with your instincts but try to judge the reaction quickly.

If it is you who has lost someone, I don't have any magic I'm afraid. I fall into the 'time is a great healer' camp. I would recommend a book that I've included at the end of the chapter about emotional healing. Do take some time off if it was someone close and give yourself some time to adjust. As far as your patients go, remember to be extra vigilant when you return to work and double check things.

Moving house

It is said that moving house rates as high as divorce and bereavement as an inducer of stress. I have pondered why that might be. I think it is influenced by whether you have chosen to move house or it has been forced upon you by other life changes.

It can be very challenging to live out of boxes and not be able to find anything. It can take a lot of adjustment when your home, the place where you should feel safe and secure, is different. The light switches are not familiar nor the toilets nor the bath nor how to work the heating nor where the fridge is. Activities of daily living become slightly uncertain. It is this shift of familiar to unfamiliar in the simply everyday things that I think contributes significantly to the stress of moving, not just the boxes. If you have moved any distance you may also need to shop somewhere new, adjust to new schools for your family and a new job, and establish new friendships.

All the previous advice applies about managing your stress levels and keeping patients safe.

Friendships and free time

There will be some who prefer a small close-knit group of friends whilst others prefer larger groups of more superficial friends. Some find it easy to make friends and for others it is a real challenge that can be quite daunting.

I think we face high pressure in healthcare. Not only can the throughput be incredibly high and the cognitive workload of the complexity of the situations be enormous, but on top of all of that is the emotional workload. When we are trying to help people who are ill or dying, especially if we cannot produce a positive outcome despite our best efforts, it has an emotional impact on us. It should not ever become something we get used to. If we harden, we lose our compassion, which is the very thing that probably took us to that role in the beginning. If we are to cope with this emotional rollercoaster, we need a support network.

I would like you to spend a couple of moments thinking about who you go to when you have seen something disturbing or emotionally draining. I hope you will have some supportive colleagues with whom you can have a chat. I hope one day, in my nirvana vision of healthcare, you will have a daily debrief so that all of this gets talked about and we all feel supported. I hope that there will be plenty of provision of coaches and mentors and counselling and access to a psychologist and sufficient occupational health but as yet, this is not currently in place (although some of us are trying to change that!).

But at home and outside, I want you to have a good network of fun and friends. When was the last time that you really laughed out loud (not the text-speak version but actually did it)? Are you able to leave your work behind you? What do you do with your spare time? If you have good friends, how often do you see them?

Whilst for some of you who have a secure friendship network and plenty of hobbies you can skip to the next bit, for others this may be a worth a few moments of thinking time.

What are you interested in that isn't work? If you have time, write a list, if not count them on your fingers. How many are there? Which of them are you currently doing and how often? Is there anything new you would like to try? How might you make the time? What would be the first step of finding out more about it?

If all the things that you do are solitary, what else might you consider that would get you meeting people?

If you have lots of friends but you don't see them enough, what are you going to do about that?

I want you to invest time and energy into your work–life balance. I am even going to mention the words exercise and fresh air.

Car parking

Whoever would have thought that when I set out to improve patient safety, patient experience, and the working lives of staff, I would be talking about the car parks!

159

I am going to focus predominantly on hospital car parks. I naïvely assumed that this topic might have been something locally relevant, but I hadn't realized that it was quite widespread. It sounds relatively simple: adequate provision of parking for the users of the service, adequate provision of parking for the providers of the service, and a financial system and administration system to support the car park.

The first problem can be waiting to actually get into the car park. The next problem is finding a space, which in some hospitals can take upwards of half an hour and can actually be impossible. Add into this the time pressure of an allocated appointment time for a patient or a clinic start time for a member of staff and we are starting to trigger an emotional response. Just to increase the angst there is the financial element. For patients this may be a combination of no change, extortionate prices, or the perceived lack of caring when having to pay to come to visit a sick relative or the uncaring approach when you have a long-term condition that will require regular hospital visits. By repeatedly paying for parking over a long time frame there is the added financial burden to add to everything else.

For staff, there have been several schemes in different hospitals that have caused an emotional response. There are set rates where all the staff pay the same that are thought to be unfair by the poorer paid. There are 'percentage of salary' rates that are deemed to be unfair by the higher paid who point out that wouldn't happen in a supermarket—the prices are the same no matter who is buying things.

When you are paying and you can't find a space, this is thought to be unfair by everyone and there is also a fairly vocal expression of 'why should I have to pay to come to work anyway!' There are accusations of 'there are patients in the staff car park' and also 'there are staff in the patients' car park'.

Why am I bothering to spend time on this topic? It is a regular source of complaints from both staff and visitors like.

It is important that we try to make the patients' and relatives' time with us as easy as possible. It is hard enough to deal with illness, difficult diagnoses, or bad news without adding to people's stress levels.

From a staff perspective, I want staff to be able to focus on what is really important—our patients. I don't want our staff feeling frazzled and antagonized before they start their day.

If we try to take a solution-based approach, let's see what ideas we can come up with. If we do some 'magic wand-type' thinking we could miraculously pick up the hospital and put it in a big open space with limitless parking space. If real estate was not an issue, we could simply expand the parking area. It is true that if hospitals are not near town centres then people cannot walk to them, so we might also need a regular bus service.

If we randomly generate ideas the following suggestions are usually put forward. A park and ride option might be useful. Car pools have been suggested. A multistorey car park on what is currently a flat car park could massively increase capacity but where does the money come from? Barrier systems and swipes instead of permits are used in some places.

What would happen if it was all free? In some places the car park would fill with shoppers and there would still be nowhere to park. But I wonder if that is true everywhere? What message would it send to our staff if they didn't have to pay for their parking? What if free parking was used as incentive scheme for longer service, encouraging staff retention? Perhaps an incentive scheme for using bicycles or walking might help?

I hope with time that other technological enablers will play a role. If, for example, we could have a swipe-able bar code on a clinic letter, we could allow our patients a free car park pass.

Of course, this would generate less income but what are our priorities?

Commuting

The journey to work is also something that our groups have reported as a source of real stress. This can be due to traffic and cars, or overfilled trains and having to stand for the entire journey, or an erratic bus service filled with noisy school children.

My only offering on this topic is to consider travelling earlier, arriving at work earlier, and then having a few minutes with a tea or a coffee during which time you can let the stress of the journey be alleviated before you start your day.

Addiction to drugs or misuse of drugs

Within certain sectors of the health service we have higher rates of addiction and suicide than the general population. I have wondered whether it is the knowledge of the drugs or their availability or the stress of the jobs that contributes to this.

Over my career I have been touched by several sad stories when members of staff have taken their lives using drugs with which they are all too familiar. There were often no warning signs and those left behind felt devastated, guilty, angry, disbelief, and denial but above all, a huge sense of sadness and loss.

I am also aware of a number of cases of addiction: a couple of examples are shared here. A member of staff was found breathing in the 'laughing gas' that is used as part of an anaesthetic. Another member of staff was found to have an opioid addiction. The latter was uncovered by an anaesthetist. The anaesthetist had drawn up the drugs for the next patient (including some morphine) and left the drugs on the side in the anaesthetic room. They were meticulous in the preparation of the drugs and always labelled them in a particular way. When they returned to put the next patient to sleep, the syringe was labelled differently. They noticed. An investigation subsequently revealed there was no longer any morphine in the syringe labelled morphine. A staff member was found to have an opioid addiction. There are countless other tales of drugs that start off as being necessary (pain killers or sedatives) becoming a long-term problem. Occupational health are skilled in managing these issues, but only if you seek their help.

Addiction to alcohol

There are changing statistics associated with excess alcohol consumption. There is increased binge drinking in teenagers with larger numbers of females involved than previously. The less obvious at-risk group are amongst the middle-aged population. These people are not out on the streets, but simply enjoying a glass of wine or two or three with a meal. The problem can be that it slowly increases and the fact that it is every night. It becomes a habit, a way to wind down after a stressful day. The problem is that a bottle of red wine, if it is around 14%, can contain 10.5 units. There are six small glasses or three large ones in a bottle. If a couple have a bottle of wine each night that would be around 5 units a night each. The rough rule of thumb that a shot is 1 unit and a pint of beer is 2 units often underestimates the true number. An alco-pop is around 1.5–2 units. The current recommended upper limits *per week* are 14 units for a woman and 21 units for a man. The most recent thoughts are that you should have at least two nights with no alcohol at all.

Another thing worth considering is how long it takes for alcohol to leave your system. As a rough rule of thumb alcohol can only be removed from your system at a steady state of 1 unit per hour. That means that if you have a big night out, stay out late and consume alcohol until 1am, if you have 10 units you will still be over the limit in the morning. Not only will you be over the limit when you drive your car but also when you come to work. You might still be over the limit when you are treating your patients.

If you when you read this, it invokes in you a defensive response about the amount you drink, I would like you to think about that response. The recent thoughts are that you should have two nights (and two days) with no alcohol per week. Do you do that?

I have included a reference to the CAGE questionnaire which has been around even since I was at medical school but I think it still applies.[1] If you answer 'yes' to two of the four questions asked, the topic of your drinking needs further investigation: the letters stand for **C**ut, **A**nnoyed, **G**uilty, and **E**ye-opener. The cut question asks if you have ever thought about cutting down on the amount you are drinking. The next question enquires whether you have ever been annoyed or become defensive when people talk about how much you drink or imply you should cut down. The next question explores whether you ever have a sense of guilt about your drinking and the final one asks if you have ever had a morning drink. The morning drink can either be to get rid of a hangover or just because you wanted one in the morning. We were also advised to ask about drinking on your own as another warning sign but that is not part of the formal questions.

As you can see, the worrying signs are not related to quantities consumed, although these are of course relevant. There are no questions about being on a park bench or having alcohol out of a bottle covered with a brown paper bag. There are also no questions about late night activities after 'throwing out' time at pubs or clubs, no mention of fights, no mention of waking up somewhere unknown or with someone unknown. Alcohol can cause a whole host of problems which can be highly visible. The one I want you to be most wary of though is the stable alcoholic. The person who drifts into having a bottle of wine each night, after all, it is just a couple of glasses with dinner . . .

Nature versus nurture: the old chestnut

Your race, your gender, your sexuality, and your age all influence who you are and how you see the world. Over time you have developed a personal value system. You will have a unique set of morals which will have been influenced not only by the factors already discussed but also by the culture that you have been exposed to. I do not only mean the culture of the country where you live now or where your ancestors came from but from the micro-cultures that you have passed through. Your family, your schooling, your friendships, and your workplace experiences will have influenced your current attitudes and how you choose your behaviours. Within our workplace there are cultural norms—'how we do it around here'. These are incredibly powerful and it is sometimes difficult to swim against the tide.

We have already alluded to the analogy of personality being like an iceberg where the part below the waterline is the personality and the visible bit is the behaviour. Our personality is generally fixed by our early twenties but it cannot be used as excuse for our behaviour. Behaviour is a choice.

While some of us will have experienced challenging life events, those too cannot be used as an excuse for long-term poor behaviour. We will consider some examples of unacceptable behaviour that the staff we surveyed reported. After that we will consider the work conditions that they felt had contributed to this.

Mood

I am not particularly interested in how a psychologist might define mood, I am more interested in what it means to you. What does being in a good mood mean to you? If I was with you, how would I know you were in a good mood? Now if I was your patient or your fellow staff member, how would they know? Don't they have a right for you to behave like that the majority of the time?

For me, a good mood involves a smile on my face, a bounce in my step, a sparkle in my eye, and a feeling I can tackle anything the day throws at me. I admit that my nickname is 'Tigger' and that I am known for my positivity. For those of you where it is not a natural tendency, I am asking you to work on it.

I have already alluded to the impact a 'mood hoover' can have on a room. There can be lots of ideas and a lovely buzz in a room until the 'mood hoover' arrives and sucks the enthusiasm from the room. I would like you to join with me to help me 'ban the mood hoover' in the NHS.

I realize we are not superhuman. I have had some challenging life events and periods of my life when I have been much more of an Eeyore than a Tigger. It can be a learnt behaviour to put a positive spin on things. I have certainly not mastered it all the time.

Do you need to change? Could you be impacting on your patients or other staff or at home with your mood? If you aren't sure where to start, a smile is a good first step, no matter how clichéd that may sound.

Unpicking things that affect your mood may also be useful. What are your emotional triggers? What frustrates you?

For me, I am much less tolerant when I am hungry and so if I can feel I'm being grumpy I have learnt to ask myself as a first port of call, 'Am I hungry?' I am also more likely to be grumpy with a lack of sleep or coffee. On a bad day, chocolate helps to elevate my mood. Interacting with some people lowers my mood. Certain behaviours in others lower my mood, for example, I don't like laziness, indecision, rudeness, and bullying. Micro-managers frustrate me as they fail to understand that by empowering their staff, they will be happier and more productive. These are a fraction of the things I have learnt about myself.

Learning about you is the essential first step. How well do you understand *your*self?

What are your triggers and how can you tackle them earlier to stop the negative mood from kicking in?

Self-direction

Do you know where you going in life? How in control of that decision do you feel?

How does your current work role sit with that direction?

For some, you may have made it as far as you want to go. For others there may be a predefined ladder that you are climbing with clear transitions and hurdles to tackle along the way. For others, there will be much more uncertainty. Some will have little say in their future as it is decided by the financial state of the institution. Others are bored or understimulated but aren't sure how to dismount from the treadmill.

How confident you are in your role also plays a part. For some, it may be 'same old, same old' but beware as a monotonous routine can lead to complacency. Complacency can also rear its head in the realm of overconfidence. Confidence is a tricky balance: too little and people will not trust that you know what you are doing; too much and the next error will be just around the corner. Overconfidence and not understanding one's limitations are two of the qualities that worry me most in a trainee with regards to safety.

How you feel in your role will affect how much you embrace it, how motivated you are to achieve things, the level of interest that you give to performing tasks, and how you are perceived by others. Job satisfaction feeds into self-esteem and self-confidence. One of the positive influences in self-esteem can be the feeling of being valued. How valued do you feel in your current role?

Is it important to you that your patients/staff feel like you value them? If the answer is no, I would have to wonder why you undertake your current role.

How much do you do to contribute to others feeling valued?

I think there are a number of ways that we can make sure our staff feel valued. For me, I think we should use the targeted praise that I have already introduced much more frequently. Not a glib, weak-willed thank you, but a hearty bit of praise that is well-thought through and personalized. I would like to see a much greater emphasis on carrot rather than stick and much more celebration of success. Even a bit of down time with a cup of tea and a cake can show some appreciation.

Ability to cope with change

As an inherent part of our personality, there are some of us that prefer a routine whilst others are happier without one. Some of us like to be organized in advance and have a plan and perhaps a list, whilst others prefer to be spontaneous and reactive. In a similar way, there are some of us that react negatively if our day suddenly has to change whilst others take that in their stride. There are some that thrive on an ever changing baseline and enjoy the adrenaline rush. For some, continual learning is an important part of any role. Look out for these individuals and celebrate their ability to adapt. They are an asset to a team.

There is no right or wrong approach, it is simply important to understand where you are on the spectrum and to understand the impact this may have in different situations. It is then possible to optimize your response and match your behaviour favourably to the setting.

Health is usually an unpredictable beast. In the setting of long-term illness there will be a fluctuating course. Even in the simplest of planned procedures, we can be faced with the unexpected situation (e.g. an anaphylactic (allergic) reaction, or a cancer we were not expecting, or some unusual anatomy). This became the daily chant of one of the senior surgeons with whom I was fortunate to work, 'Always expect the unexpected!'. We need to be adaptable. We cannot plan for the eventualities of each case. We cannot plan for the number of cases when emergency or urgent cases are added. We must therefore devise systems that inherently cope with change.

On top of that there is innovation. We want to strive to improve our care and our outcomes. We have new equipment, new drugs, new techniques, and new treatments. These are positive changes but how are we sharing them and ensuring that we take others with us?

We work with a continuously changing political baseline. We are pawns in a vote-winning agenda. This results in what feels like an almost continuous stream of restructuring. This results in a 'change weary' workforce.

As far as change goes there are several approaches: the ostrich 'head-in-the-sand' denial approach; sulking; increased noise and in-fighting; banging your head against the change; the voice of doom ('it will never work', 'we've tried it all before'); and then there are those that cope.

Are you familiar with the following?

Cliché alert: we need to move to a place where change is how we do business! I'm not saying that the words are the ones I would choose, but the sentiment is. We need to have enough slack built into the system so that we can continue to adjust and adapt to the challenges that are thrust upon us. Part of this is capacity planning so that we are not overstretched all the time.

We need to be able to learn every day. There will be small errors/inefficiencies every day. We need to look for them. We need to talk about them at a daily chat (debrief) at the end of every day (or night!). We need to think about how we will stop ourselves making that same mistake again. On a good day it will simply be a tweak in efficiency to make the service even better (icing the cake). On a bad day, we may all need to sit down and perhaps fill in a SHEEP sheet and use it as a basis for a learning conversation. We may need to support each other through some difficult emotional 'stuff' along the way. We need to replace blame with a balanced ownership and responsibility for change and continuous improvement.

When we start to look for improvements every day, we will have achieved the learning culture that we are striving to create.

What are you going to do differently today?

Preparation and expectations

How adaptable we are and how we react to the spontaneous changes that can come our way, leads us on to preparation. How prepared do you like to be before you tackle something? For some, it may be that you would naturally repeat something and perfect it prior to trying it out for real. Others are more prepared to 'wing it'.

If we consider a couple of surgical examples we can contrast a couple of very typecast cases. If there is a delicate eye case which is being performed with a microscope with a surgical thread (suture) that is so fine you can hardly see it, it might be reasonable to hope that the surgeon has practised tying those knots over and over again so that they can achieve it with precision in a repeatable way. If a patient has been knifed and has multiple stab wounds throughout their abdomen, it may not be possible to rehearse for what might be found. Just when things seem to be under control there could be an unexpected extra bit of damage that starts bleeding as the blood pressure has been restored to normal levels. Different personalities will cope differently in different settings. Do you know where your strengths lie?

If you are a 'planner' and you find yourself in the deep end, you can feel unprepared. This can result from two broad categories of events. There are completely unexpected events: the stabbing victim. There are other events which can be anticipated but there is a lack of information flow across a department or an organization, this can result in the same outcome: an unexpected event. For those who are not planners who leave things to the last minute, I urge you to consider the impact this may have on a 'planner'.

It is also really important to check when you are planning things with others to check that you have a shared understanding. It is useful to double check that you have achieved a shared mental model. Something along the lines of, 'Let me check I've got this clear in my mind . . . ' and describe it, clarifying the time scale, should help. Then write it down together and give everyone a copy. It is not my intention to use this as a back covering exercise: this is to generate a shared direction.

The same can be true when we are planning something with people: a procedure, a treatment, the management plan, the next clinic visit. Be honest about what is realistic. I would always only promise something I could definitely deliver, erring on the side of caution. When running an unpredictable emergency theatre list, I explain that I cannot say what time the surgery will take place. I suggest a time slightly later than when I think it will be but explain that the sickest patients are done first. I promise them we will get to them as quickly as we can and we discuss a plan to manage their pain/sickness/symptoms in the meantime. I find this open approach is met with understanding. My personal belief is that the problems start when we haven't told people what to expect or if we have told them something that we cannot deliver. It is the failure to meet expectations of both patients and staff that causes disappointment and resentment and possibly frustration (see Example 6.2).

How good are you at being realistic and honest when you are explaining things so that people are fully prepared for what they face?

Example 6.2 A mismatch of explanation and expectations

A fit 40-something female bravely faced the news of a diagnosis of rectal cancer. She coped valiantly with chemotherapy and radiotherapy, with major surgery, with a colostomy, and with yet more chemotherapy.

After 9 months of treatment, she went for a scan and was given the all clear. There was great celebration.

Now at last, she could have her reversal and get back to living her life. The day arrived. The operation went uneventfully.

What, however, was not at all clear was that she would have to be near a toilet at all times. As all the storage facilities of the previous bowel had been removed, the new bowel was not educated to perform its new function. Diarrhoea would happen frequently with no warning and it would mean she couldn't leave the house.

This conversation had not been covered by the hospital staff. There was no preparation for this bombshell. There has still been no conversation about how long this might go on for: a week, a month, forever?

Letting someone find out about these side effects on their own when they are at home is surely not the best way to handle the situation.

She had spent 9 months looking forward to getting back to normal. The surgeons had made it all sound like a walk in the park. It has not been one.

It is time for honesty and fuller explanations.

How you are influenced by your work

We have already considered some of the ways our home life and our past experiences can have an impact on how we are at work. Our work itself can also impact on how we work.

We have already alluded to the fact that an argument or conflict can result in someone being distracted afterwards and hence there is a period when an error is more likely. It can also impact on anyone who was present or even peripherally involved. It is one of many things that will lower moral. Try to speak up early before things become a problem and resolve it in an adult–adult approach (see 'Conflict resolution' in Chapter 3).

We have already discussed how important it is that we use praise and show our appreciation so that our staff feel valued. A positive outlook will lift a room. Think how you can banish the 'mood hoover' and not allow a 'whinge fest'. Replace this with a positive way of eliciting ideas for improvement and ongoing change. Then more praise! Team working is important; we need to invest time and effort to develop our teams. We need to be inclusive and help people feel like they fit in and belong. All of these things will help raise moral and increase job satisfaction.

Cliché alert: happy staff means happy patients.

We need to take seriously the impact that working over our hours might have on us if it happens over a longer time frame. We need to take some rest breaks. When we are away from work we need to leave it behind us.

We need to understand the impact of shift work, especially night shifts. We need to think about when we should be more error aware and how we will modify our behaviour accordingly, introducing double checking or commentating (talking out loud) on the task we are performing.

We need to understand that time pressure and urgency of the situation will have an impact on our decision-making. It is a time to involve more people views and watch for a fixation error. Remember to keep asking, 'what are we missing?' or 'what else could this be?'. There is also more chance of error in times of high workload.

Key points from Chapters 1–6

- We all make mistakes. We can get better at anticipating them with practice. Are you looking at how to avoid your next one?

- We need to embed an open culture.

- There should be an inquisitive approach to error that seeks out the learning and shares it: the learning culture.

- The new error checklist—the SHEEP sheet—helps gather more information following an actual event or a nearly event. The SHEEP sheet can be used for trend analysis.

- Information flow across an organization can be achieved using a brief/debrief model using Debbie's Diamond.

- Systems errors are commonly part of the holes in the Swiss cheese and should feature in the solutions for improved safety.

- Things are not always what they seem: avoid assumption.

- 'What am I missing here?' is a healthy question to keep asking.

- If the hierarchy is too steep, the team will not feel able to challenge the leader when they are making a mistake. We all make mistakes.

- If there is a flat hierarchy, no natural leader emerges, ask the question, 'Who's leading?'

- Followership is a much overlooked and important skill to have. This can involve being assertive enough to speak up if things are about to go wrong.

- We will all push someone else's buttons. We can't change the other person, only ourselves.

- We need to become more aware of how we are impacting on others (increase our self-awareness). This might begin with knowing our preferred learning style, team role, and our personality type (MBTI).

- Once we know who we are more likely to 'clash' with, we can try and blend in a bit better (self-management) to avoid conflict.

- If we do end up in conflict we will behave in an assertive way (this is completely different from aggressive although the terms are often mis-used) and aim to find a win–win situation.

- A good leader will be able to switch to using four different leaderships styles when appropriate and will avoid micro-management or pacesetting. (This pacesetting style currently dominates the NHS in both clinical and non-clinical leaders.)

- Remember when giving feedback and praise:

  - Situation Behaviour Impact Change or Continue.

- Knowing where everything is and having it laid out in a logical, clearly marked way not only makes it more efficient but it makes it safer.

- Standardizing the layout of clinical areas decreases errors.

- If you are doing a transfer, plan and plan some more.

- Try not to interrupt others. If you are interrupted yourself, start the task again if you can and watch for errors.

- Try not to stand over patients in their beds and talk down to them. Always imagine how they might be feeling.

- SBAR—situation, background, assessment, recommendation/request— is good for handovers of information especially on the phone.

- 'Active identification' needs to become standard practice with all drug administration and before any procedure and before any clinical interaction.

- It is possible to design equipment to eliminate layers of cheese and to decrease the chance of error.

- Being adequately trained on a piece of equipment is essential. Subsequent skill maintenance is also essential, particularly if the kit is used infrequently.

- Training with simulation offers an alternative for acquiring and maintaining skills.

- If your physiological needs are not being met leaving you hungry, thirsty, tired, or in need of the toilet, you are more likely to make a mistake.

- The 'two-breath' technique can help manage your stress levels in a crisis.

- We will all suffer life events at some point, be careful how these can impact on you at work.

- We have stressful jobs. Don't be afraid to ask for support. Those around you will need support too.

Reference

1. Ewing JA. 'Detecting alcoholism: the CAGE questionnaire'. *Journal of the American Medical Association* 1984;252:1905–7.

Potentially useful reading material

Thomas A. Harris. *I'm OK – You're OK*. London: Arrow Books, 2012.

Susan Jeffers. *Feel the Fear and Do It Anyway*. London: Arrow Books, 1993.

Nancy Kline. *Time to Think*. London: Cassell, 1998.

Gael Lindenfield. *The Emotional Healing Strategy*. London: Penguin, 2008.

Mark Williams and Danny Penman. *Mindfulness*. London: Piatkus, 2011.

7

Communication: face to face is best

It is the province of knowledge to speak and it is the privilege of wisdom to listen

Oliver Wendell Holmes (1809–1894)
The Poet at the Breakfast-Table (1872), chapter 10

Introduction

I want to break communication down into five types:

1. **Information transfer:** person to person, i.e. one person has some information and then needs to successfully ensure that the other person understands it and takes it away with them.

2. **Information flow:** when information is needed to be transferred across groups of people or departments of organizations.

3. **Social chat:** a much less structured format and not something I will be covering.

4. **Dealing with distress.**

5. **Debriefing after an event:** a supportive, coaching style, learning conversation.

This chapter focuses on only one of these: the first one. This is what seems to go wrong in so many cases. We have already talked about information flow, dealing with distress, and we have touched on debriefing (I will devote considerable time to this in the second book). I'm sure most of you probably mastered the chatting bit in primary school.

Have you ever spent time really thinking about how good you are at communicating and how you could be even better?

If you have time, get a pen and paper and try Exercise 7.1.

Exercise 7.1 What does communication look like?

I want you to have a go at trying to draw the process of communication.

By communication in this context I mean face to face, one person to one person. I want you to think about transferring a piece of information rather than a chat.

This is distinct from what we have already called large-scale information flow or organizational communication.

I want you to try and work out how many steps there are in successful communication. Only when we fully understand a process can we start to think about how we might improve it.

Put it aside and we will come back to it.

You may have already established whether you are an 'E' or an 'I' on the Myers Briggs type indicator. A famous example of the former said something along the lines of, 'how will I know what I am thinking until I hear it?'. For some, there is the clichéd tendency to talk first and think later. This first part of your personality type will affect how you communicate as will your preference for either big picture versus detail and whether you tend to go with your head or your heart.

So before we start to talk there is some brain activity where, either briefly, or with great thought, we prepare the words.

Even before the words come out there are lots of others things at play. There are the influences of life experiences to date (culture, the language you speak, age, gender, etc.). There are the influences of work (time pressure, work load, background noise levels, hierarchy, role, etc.). There are the influences from how your day has gone so far (car parking, woken up by the children, recent life event, mood, hungry, etc.). There is whether you have met the person before and how that went (first meeting or history, get on well, had a row last time you met). Then there are perceptions; we will explore this but for now start with the premise that you are more likely to see or to hear what you are expecting to see or hear.

Before we even open our mouths there is also the body language that has already happened. The facial expression, the eye contact, the posture, the movement (both speed and style), the way we are dressed, and the assumptions we are already making.

Imagine this is an interaction with a patient and a member of staff. Imagine the patient is in a bed on a ward. As the staff member approaches, the patient already has an inkling of whether the staff member looks rushed or relaxed and in control. Who would you like to be looked after by?

The staff member may have looked at whether the patient is in pain, whether they are breathing quickly, whether they are fully alert, whether they are pale, whether they are attached to lots of drips, and they may have focused on whether they seem anxious or not.

Whilst studies have disagreed about how much of communication is non-verbal, I usually go with a mid-range value of around 70% (range 55–80%).

I am not of the school of thought that certain body language always means the same thing. I think there are personal and cultural differences. I would like you to become self-aware with regard to body language. When are you open or closed? How much is the right amount of eye contact for a situation? Are you fiddling with something? Do you really look like you are listening? When you are in a meeting, are you ever on your laptop or texting or using some other form of electronic device? It could be that you are actually taking notes, but how else might it be interpreted?

As an aside for a moment I would like you to cast your mind back to the last time you listened to someone who was really boring you. (Perhaps you can recall a lecturer, a school teacher, a news programme, or an interview with a minor 'celeb'.) What was it that contributed to the boredom factor? For a reasonable proportion of you, I would expect that a monotonous drone will have featured. It is this change in tone of voice that also contributes to successful communication. If we take away the variety of tones, we are far more likely to disengage and switch off from the conversation. Tone, pace, and pitch probably contributes around a further 25% (range 20–38%) to successful communication.

And yes, the more able mathematicians will have already surmised that the words themselves therefore represent a mere 5% of the communication. Studies vary slightly so forgive me a few per cent here and there.

This serves as a reminder of something we covered in an earlier chapter, that it is very difficult to communicate successfully by either text or email and only marginally easier by phone. Beware! I recommend that you stick to the 'three-line rule' and use the written media of text and email for simple concepts only. If you can't say it in three lines, go and see them face to face instead. On the phone, we should be standardizing the way our transfer of information takes place. There are a number of tools available to help structure a conversation so that the chances of it happening successfully are increased. SBAR and RSVP are two of the common ones. It is important for an organization to choose one tool. I am going to use SBAR for my examples (SBAR stands for Situation, Background, Assessment, Recommendation/Request).

Just before we start that I'm going to introduce you to something that I informally call the 'funnel technique'. Rather than information arriving in any order we are going to think about the big picture versus the detail. See Exercise 7.2: How to funnel.

Exercise 7.2 How to funnel

I need you to enter into an imaginary Christmas spirit and we have reached the part of the day when we start to play games.

You will need two pieces of paper and a pen.

The rules are that I have been given the name of an object and a list of words that I am not allowed to say. You are going to draw my object.

Draw a square. Draw four more squares and a rectangle. Half way down the rectangle, draw a very small rectangle in the opposite orientation from the first one. On the top of the square is a triangle.

In a Rolf Harris moment, I now enthusiastically enquire whether you can 'tell what it is yet?' with an appalling attempt at an Australian accent. Can you?

Please take the second piece of paper. Let's try that again but with some funnelling!

Take the second piece of paper. Do not draw any of the parts until asked to do so.

Before you draw anything, I'm going to give you an overview. This object is a dwelling. It is something that we drew as children. It is drawn without a ruler and has a childlike feel to it. It would be a classic two-up and two-down. The paper should be landscape. Taking up most of the page (about 1/2 of it) and positioned centrally; draw a large square. Now stop drawing again.

As we don't want the rain to enter our dwelling it has something on top. It is a triangle that is symmetrical and it sits right on top of the square. The height takes the building to within one finger breadth of the top of the paper. It doesn't overhang off the sides of the square. If you are happy please draw the triangle. If you are not happy, please re-read this paragraph to check the details and then attempt the drawing.

Every such dwelling needs some things to let the light come in and for the occupants to see out. There are four of them. They are all squares. They are symmetrically placed with two on the first storey of the building and two on the ground level. Please draw the four squares.

There is an entrance to the property. It opens and closes. It is currently closed. It is a rectangle which sits in between the panes of glass on the lower storey. Its height is slightly higher than the panes of glass. It goes to the bottom of the main square. It does not have a visible handle. It does, however, have a letterbox. This is a small rectangle slightly below the middle of the main rectangle and it goes across (not up and down). Please draw the two rectangles.

Please put your two drawings alongside each other. How do they compare?

Now please look at Figure 7.1: My drawing and Figure 7.2: Funnel.

Now that you have hopefully grasped the concept of the funnel, I want to reintroduce at this stage the structured communication tool SBAR (see Example 7.1). Again we start with a big picture opener—what is the point of this conversation? This is then followed by honing in on the detail. It is all done using a standardized framework.

BIG PICTURE

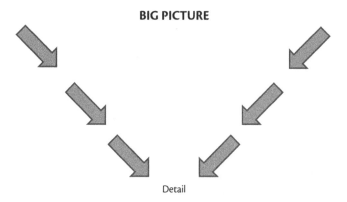

Detail

Figure 7.2 Funnel.

Example 7.1 SBAR communication tool

Situation: State your name, where you are, and what/who you are calling about, (the big picture).

Background: Briefly describe history and any important information.

Assessment: Give your assessment of the patient/situation. If relevant, include ABCDE assessment and an early warning score (e.g. ViEWS/ PEWS/MEWS).

Recommendations: Request help.

Be clear about what you want.

Put a time frame on your request (now/within 30 minutes/today/next week).

Ask what you can do in the meantime.

Reproduced with permission from SBAR (Situation, Background, Assessment, Recommendation), Quality and Service Improvement Tools, Copyright © NHS Institute for Innovation and Improvement 2008, available from <http://www.institute.nhs.uk/quality_and_service_improvement_tools/ quality_and_service_improvement_tools/quality_and_service_improvement_tools_for_the_nhs.html>.

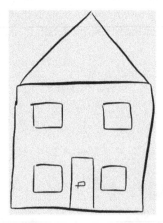

Figure 7.1 My drawing.

Using this tool, I would like you to try a fictitious exercise. There is a 'wood from the trees' element to it. I have written an example of a 'bad' day when things are not going quite to plan. I would like you to read through the scenario (see Box 7.1). Now copy out the blank template (Figure 7.3) onto a piece of paper. Now re-read Box 7.1 and fill in all the sections on your blank template on your paper.

I hope that you can now see that the tool can be used not only for handing over the information for one patient but for a whole situation. If I had my way, I would have an SBAR sticker on every phone throughout the whole NHS. I would have all telephone conversations following the SBAR format within an organization and for referrals from primary to secondary or for discharges in the opposite direction and so on . . . !

Box 7.1 Fictitious bad day

The bed manager system is not working. I need to pick up the children from school after work. It is 2.30pm. We have no beds available on Intensive Care. Is it time to trigger the escalation system? I am hungry and tired as I haven't eaten or had a break all shift. There are two very sick patients in the Recovery Unit who have been assessed and need to be transferred to Intensive Care. I can't find the policy with regards to triggering the escalation system. Each very sick patient needs one nurse. I find the Ops Manager intimidating. It is raining. My mum's car is in the garage being fixed so she couldn't help with a school pick up today. I am craving chocolate. My pager keeps going off. My shift finishes in half an hour. The internal IT system has failed. I am on Intensive Care. There is currently a shortage of nurses. I couldn't find a parking space this morning. There are no porters available. There are two patients in the Emergency Department who have been assessed and are now waiting to be moved to Intensive Care. I was up in the night as one of my children had a high temperature. I wonder how they are and if my mum is coping? It is possible to stop theatre to free up more staff by triggering the escalation system. All four patients who are outliers are already intubated and ventilated (on breathing machines). I had an argument with my partner this morning before I came to work because he forgot to put the bins out. How mindless is that! I must apologize to him later. Today is Tuesday. I am a senior nurse/senior doctor/senior manager (choose) on intensive care responsible for solving this crisis. The coffee machine is broken, I love coffee. I have to make a phone call to relay relevant parts of this information to the Ops Manager.

Let us go back to considering what communication is often considered to be and the drawing you did for what does communication look like.

I want to focus further on this idea of information transfer rather than a chat or helping someone in distress or debriefing them after a difficult event.

We will consider a really simple piece of information. We will imagine that we are supposed to be at a meeting together on Friday this week but I need to change the time from 9am to 10am. We will assume you are free at 10 am and that would be OK. It is only the two of us that are meeting. This should surely be a really easy process to get that information across.

We will assume I have just bumped into you in the corridor and we have already said hello.

How many steps are there? A simple five-step model is shown in Figure 7.4.

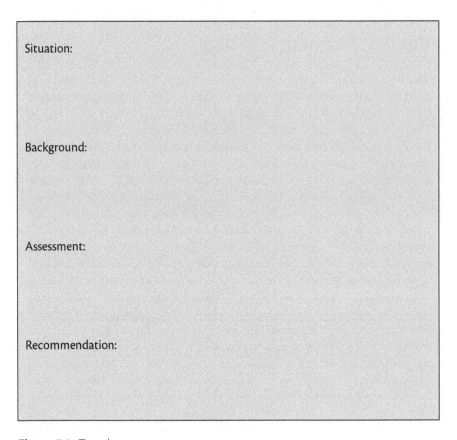

Situation:

Background:

Assessment:

Recommendation:

Figure 7.3 Template.

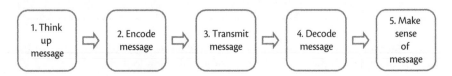

Figure 7.4 Five-step model.

This is a fairly standard approach to drawing communication but for me it has missing steps and it is far too simple. It doesn't explain why it is different every time and all of the complexities. Neither does it explain how to improve it. Person 1 thinks up what they want to say. They then change these thoughts into words (encode). The second person hears the words and decodes them (translates them into thoughts to make sense of them). There is nothing to represent clarification and no final confirmation that the message has been accurately transmitted and understood. There is no mention of preconceptions and assumptions. There is no mention of non-verbal communication.

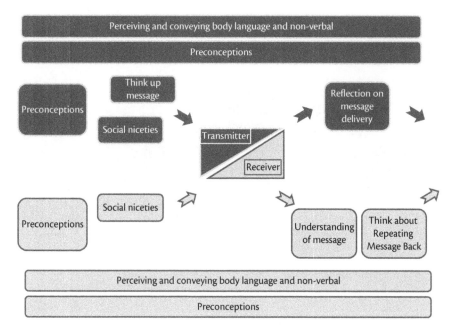

Figure 7.5 Face-to-face communication model.

I am going to add in a few more steps. In the flow diagram there are two people involved. I have coloured them differently (see Figure 7.5).

Figure 7.5 builds on the basics but starts to add in some more complexities. But in addition to this phase, there should be another phase which I have included in Figure 7.6.

As we approach each other we start to form ideas about what might happen next. These are based on who we are, our past experiences, our values, our personalities, what sort of day we have had up to that point, what life events we are currently living through, how well we know the other person, how was it when we last met them, etc. I am going to imply that these result in what I'm going to refer to as our preconceptions and assumptions. The other person in the interaction will also have their past experiences, their values, their personality, a day that will influence their mood and behaviour, life events, and perhaps a completely different recall of the last meeting. I am again going to package the end product of all of these under the heading of preconceptions and assumptions. I think these assumptions and preconceptions have a large part to play in the initial interaction, but I think they also influence every stage of the communication process.

As the preconceptions and assumptions are already beginning, so is the non-verbal communication. The posture, the speed of the approach, the amount of eye contact, a smile (or not) and whether it is returned, a hand shake or a

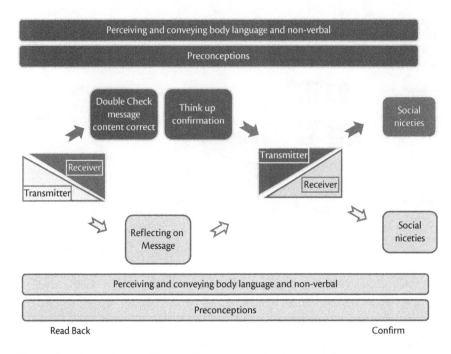

Figure 7.6 Second part of face-to-face communication model.

more familiar touch or peck on the cheek will all colour the beginning of the communication.

There are usually some culturally influenced social niceties (the weather, the journey to work, or if you know each other better how the children are) which start the conversation.

If we imagine then the simple message of the changed meeting time to use as our example. We think of the concept of the message. There is then a coupled process of transmission and receiving. The speaker needs to explain clearly using clean language matched to the person with whom they are talking. The listener needs to be active in their listening. The processes are simultaneous with only the tiniest of lag times rather than the sequential steps by which they are traditionally represented. I have shown both parties to be contributing to this process as it is coupled or shared.

Once the information has been heard by the receiver, they convert this auditory information into thoughts and process the information.

At this point in most traditional models communication is deemed to have taken place. For me, it is that assumption, the assumption that communication has been successful, that causes a lot of the problems.

For me, the process should continue. The receiver should think about repeating the message back to check they have it correctly. In the meantime, the transmitter of the message will be having a think about what they said and watching all the non-verbal communication about how it was received. The subsequent steps are seen in Figure 7.6.

The roles are briefly reversed. The original receiver now transmits. They repeat back what they think they heard (read back). The original transmitter then confirms that is the correct interpretation of the message. Throughout each of these processes there is continuous perception and conveying of non-verbal communication by both parties. All of the preconceptions and assumptions are also at play.

The conversation would probably finish with some sort of social niceties and a good bye.

With this two-part model I think it is more obvious why miscommunication is commonplace. It is really quite a complex interaction but we take it for granted that we can do it. Most of us in healthcare might even assume we are naturally good communicators . . . How good are you?

Take a moment to imagine a chance meeting with a friend. Imagine we script a conversation between the two of you. Now rewind and substitute another of your friends into the scene. Imagine that you start with exactly the same words and you are following the same script. Would the conversation be the same? What would be different?

I would imagine the body posture, the facial expressions, the tone and the inflections of the voices, the use of silence or pause, the rate of speech, and the hand gestures would all be different. We have already established that these represent the lion share of communication. It would not be a huge leap of faith therefore to imagine that the meaning would be interpreted differently. In a social setting, it may not be a serious consequence if there is a miscommunication. In healthcare, however, it is vital that we improve our communication as it is one of the highest contributory factors in error.

How might you need to communicate differently to make you safer?

We have already discussed that the greatest proportion of communication comes from non-verbal communication. We have said the next most important factors are due to tone of voice, pattern of speech, speed of speech and intonation, and the use of pause and silence. And this left only a small proportion of the responsibility with the words. But let us now think a bit more about those words.

If we play with written communication in the first instance, I would like you to read Figure 7.7.

Aoccdrnig to rscheearch at Cmabrigde Uinervtisy, it deson't mttaer in waht oredr the leettrs are, the olny iprmoetnt tihng is taht the frist and lsat ltteer are in the rghit pclae. The rset can be a toatl mses and you can sitll raed it fialry eaisly. Tihs is bcuseae we do not raed ervey lteter, but the wrod as a wlohe.

Figure 7.7 How we interpret written information is surprising.

Communication with patients: choosing the words

In a clinical setting we need to choose language that our patients understand. How we pitch the conversation depends on the background knowledge of the people, their culture, values, intelligence, their emotional state, and how all of these things interact with our own equivalent factors. This is why it is so tricky to get it right every time. The initial conversation needs to try to grasp these influencing factors: a sort of background check. There is a balancing act between pitching at the right level and not being patronizing or condescending. It needs to be matched with an appropriate mood and demeanour. Whilst I fully sign up to the good old cliché that a smile costs nothing, in healthcare settings, when someone is seriously ill or worse, there are times when a smile is not the right approach.

As the conversation is progressing we are constantly looking for clues about how the information is being received. We need to check understanding as we progress. We need to watch body language and facial expression. We need to listen. We need to be comfortable with the use of silence.

It is important that we check that we have successfully transferred the information across and not just assume that because we said it, we have communicated successfully. We need to focus on the read back and confirmation parts of the process which are often either ignored or brushed over. Remembering that only a fraction of the information we deliver is taken on board, giving a written summary of the key points for people to take away with them is useful.

If you are expecting to have a difficult conversation: prepare for it in advance and practise the words you might use; rehearse.

In summary

> **Background check . . . deliver message . . . check understanding . . . and repeat.**

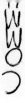

Alternative summary

Tell them what you are going to tell them . . . tell them . . . then tell them what you told them. But check they understood it!

Communication with other staff: choosing the words

We have seen that written words can be interpreted even with the letters jumbled up (see Figure 7.7). However, if we think about words when we are speaking, we need to choose them very carefully. We need to use 'clean language' that is not ambiguous.

There are certain words that are culturally acceptable within different subcultures of the NHS but which completely alienate other subcultures. I believe these change within quite short time frames but I include a list (in Box 7.2) of what I consider to be current danger phrases that will often result in 'skying eyes', sighs, or even 'tuts'.

Box 7.2 Phrases that press buttons

- Blue sky thinking, silo thinking
- A journey/a path/pathway
- Personal growth/growing someone
- A vision/mission statement
- Thinking outside the box
- With respect . . .
- Work with me here
- I have heard you, I hear what you are saying
- Going forward, pre-prepare and forward planning, forward thinking
- This time it is different
- My door is open
- Cascading
- Joined up thinking, keep me in the loop, close the loop, run with this

- We need to be proactive on this one
- We are all on same team here, we need to pull in the same direction
- It's not you, it's me
- We are looking for the win–win
- Let's touch base/hook up
- We have the making of a perfect storm
- Push back/challenge.

I'm sure the list is endless and changes fairly rapidly. I think it is culturally dependent. I have heard clinicians moan about 'management speak' and the managers moan about medical terminology. I think we need to be aware of each other's buttons and to try not to press them. We need to have in our minds that we should tailor-make our conversation to our audience. It is not about how you would like to be spoken to, but about how the receiver would like to be spoken to. This brings us back to the concept of emotional intelligence. With a greater amount of awareness, we can better match our style to our audience.

We have talked about words and phrases to avoid but we haven't yet covered topics that are safe and frameworks for how to put them in place. I find the onion model useful to illustrate this.

If you imagine a typical conversation in an NHS setting, what might be the first things that are discussed? Perhaps you might open with a comment about the weather or maybe the car parking or perhaps the journey in? The conversation starts at a safe superficial level in the realm of the ritual and the cliché. I think the obsession with the weather is particularly British. I am sure there will be cultural differences with these classic openers.

We might then move on to the next layer of the onion: the facts and figures. 'How many have we got booked in to clinic/theatre list today? What are our staffing levels? What is our current waiting time? How many have we got waiting for beds?'

We may venture slightly further depending on how well we know each other, our personality combinations, our shared knowledge and values into the realms of the next layer: the ideas and beliefs. 'Any thoughts on why that is happening? How could we improve on that? What might be the next steps?'.

A good leader and a good follower will probe a bit deeper: the feelings and emotions. This layer is not traditionally very British at all. It doesn't fit easily with a stiff upper lip and carry on regardless. It also doesn't fit so easily with some personality types. If we take the classic ISTJ (the most common group Myers Briggs type in an executive or board room), they are unlikely to be naturally in touch with discussing feelings. These are some of the shifts in behaviour we are going to need to produce truly great leaders and perhaps to recapture some of the missing compassion that gets lost in hitting financial targets. 'How did you feel when that happened? How is everyone coping? You seem upset. What impact will this change have on you?'

If you fall into that category (grey suit and ISTJ and yes, my tongue may be sitting in my check to see if I can get a reaction), I would urge you to consider how you are going to rise to that challenge. The evidence is out there to suggest the change is beneficial.

There is a final layer of the onion: the layer which we will not share at work. The topics which fall into this category will be different for each of us.

What might be your first step?

We have looked the idea that there are some words which might be inflammatory. An awareness of these is useful. We would like to use something that is referred to as 'clean language'. This is language which is not ambiguous and it is easily understood. The language we use needs to take account of many personal factors of the speaker and the listener such as age, gender, culture, mother tongue, emotional overlay, intelligence, and so on. The speaker should attempt to tailor-make it for the receiver taking all of these factors into account but without being patronizing. In reality no matter how good we think we are at communicating this task is very complex. The receiver has a responsibility too, to clarify and confirm understanding. We must remember that the listener may only take away a small proportion of what has been discussed. We may need to backup what we have tried to convey with written information that can be taken away to be digested over time.

Each of us at some time will be the one that presses someone else's buttons. It is helpful to receive this feedback openly. Try to avoid becoming defensive. Remember that within a relationship or interaction you can only modify yourself and your own behaviour. You cannot change the person or the behaviour of the person you are dealing with.

Berne observed patterns of behaviour when he watched individuals interact. He matched the behaviour to a simple concept of three states with which we are all familiar: parent, child, and adult. The idea of 'transactional analysis' is to notice when you are being pulled into either child or parent modes and to try to stay in adult mode. Examples of parental phrases might be, 'You must do it this way . . .', 'Grow up!', 'Haven't you finished that yet?'. While the petulant child mode may be more along the lines of, 'I'm not doing it!', 'Stop hassling me!'. If the person with whom we are talking slips into parent, they can 'hook' our inner child. It is challenging sometimes to stay in adult mode rather than just become reactive. Having mastered self, the next step is to try and pull them back to adult–adult. If we stay with a relationship where the communication is let's say 'less than ideal', the first thing to try to do is to modify ourselves. If we have tried this we need to move to phase 2: feedback.

I want to reiterate how to give feedback: situation, behaviour, impact and change or continue (or SBIC). Stick to things you have witnessed rather than hearsay. Think about where you are going to have the conversation, it should be somewhere private with solid walls not curtains (**situation**). Describe what you observed objectively and without emotion. Describe the **behaviour** and not the personality. Do not bring up past occurrences. Do not judge in your body language, tone or words. Describe the **impact** that it had on you when you watched it as an 'I' statement. This means starting with the word 'I'. Either 'I felt . . . ' or 'I thought . . . '. Finally ask them how they could have done it differently. If they cannot think of another way of doing it, suggest a **change** for them but it is more powerful if they come up with it themselves. If you are using the tool for praise (and please do more of this) then the last bit is to encourage them to **continue** to behave in that way.

If there is still no progress following feedback on multiple occasions then it is sometimes time to walk away or to pursue a more formal managerial route.

We have focused on how we might deliver our message. But what are we like at receiving the message?

Listening

This is a vital, but often overlooked skill. We have shared a few jokes about old-fashioned communication skills classes that used to have a formulaic approach to empathy. When delivering bad news there was a certain list of instructions, 'tilt your head, lean in, pause, and touch the patient's knee gently, with eyes glancing slightly down' . . . which would potentially make a good comedy sketch. There is no absolute way to behave that will suit all situations.

There has been a lot of interest recently in the concept of 'active listening'. Just being quiet is not enough. There should be an acknowledgement that you are listening. This might be with non-verbal cues such as a slight nod of the head or the occasional 'mmm' or 'uh, huh' or a positive affirmation. The amount of eye contact is important; enough to show that you listening but not too much. Learning to be comfortable with silence can be quite hard. A short amount of time can feel very feel very uncomfortable until you get used to it. The natural tendency is to try to fill the silence: resist this temptation: allow the person time to think or to come to terms with what has just been said.

When it comes to repeating back to someone what they have just said there a few approaches that might be useful. In a clinical, factual situation such as reading out the label on a drug bottle, then just read it back. No fancy preamble is necessary.

If you are in a conversation you need to listen hard enough to be able to achieve the following: repeating the information back in the words of the person; giving a summary of what you have heard in your own words or listening to everything and putting together a hypothesis which you can then propose. Listening to this level takes practice. It can be helpful to make a reference to which type of feedback of information you are going to use, for example: 'In my words, what I think you said was . . . '.

The human brain can only cope with around seven items in a list. So if there is more information than that, even as the receiver, try to break the information into sections. This is called chunking. For example, 'That sounds like a lot to be dealing with. Let me check I've got it all straight in my mind. What I thought you said was . . . Have I missed anything? Have I got it right?'.

Communication in a crisis

ABCDE

Assess patient and start lifesaving treatment. Do a running commentary so that everyone can follow your thinking. This not only encourages a shared mental model but it will slow you down slightly, make you clarify what you think and help manage your stress levels.

People—who?

Who have we got? What are their roles?
Who is leading? Leader commentates on thought processes and actions to encourage shared mental model.
Use ABCDE to allocate tasks and roles—matched for skills—give a running commentary of role allocation and check each person is clear.
Is someone timing and scribing?
Who is missing? How long will it take to get them here and who is going to initiate that?

What is it?

What is the diagnosis? Verbalize the emergency nature. Verbalize the diagnosis. What else could it be? What are we missing?

What are we going to do?

Verbalize the algorithm being used or pathway or treatment plan. Allocate someone to find a written down version of it to use an aide memoir. What tests do we need? What other treatment might we need?

Equipment—with what?

What equipment or drugs have we got?
What's missing that we might need? How can we get it here? Who is going to 'own' that?

Where?

Are we in the best place to deal with this?
If not, where should we be? Would it be safe to move?

Who else?

Have we thought about family?
Have we warned other services that we might need their help in the next steps?

What next?

What else should we be doing? (All members of the team are asked for suggestions.)
What are we missing here?

And review

◆ Patient—ABCDE

◆ Staff and roles

- Diagnosis and treatment plan

- Equipment

- Environment

- Family and future staff (if we are moving to different ward/theatre/hospital)

- Next steps.

Key points from Chapters 1–7

- The commonest type of mistake is poor communication but we are going to think of this as a failure of information transfer.

- By using 'read back' and clarification we can increase the chances of successful information transfer.

- We all make mistakes. We can get better at anticipating them with practice. Are you looking at how to avoid your next one?

- We need to embed an open culture. What might your first steps be to help this become a reality?

- There should be an inquisitive approach to error that seeks out the learning and shares it: the learning culture.

- How is learning shared in your organization?

- The new error checklist—the SHEEP sheet—helps gather more information following an actual event or a nearly event. The SHEEP sheet can be used for trend analysis. By looking at trends, preventative measures can be targeted.

- Information flow across an organization can be achieved using a brief/ debrief model using Debbie's diamond.

- Systems errors are commonly part of the holes in the Swiss cheese and should feature in the solutions for improved safety.

- Things are not always what they seem: avoid assumption.

- 'What am I missing here?' is a healthy question to keep asking.

- If the hierarchy is too steep, the team will not feel able to challenge the leader if they are making a mistake. We all make mistakes.

- If there is a flat hierarchy and no natural leader emerges, ask the question, 'Who's leading?'.

- Followership is a much overlooked and important skill to have. One aspect is being assertive enough to speak up if things are about to go wrong.

- We will all push someone else's buttons. We can't change the other person, only ourselves.

- We need to become more aware of how we are impacting on others (increase our self-awareness). This might begin with knowing our preferred learning style, team role and our personality type (MBTI).

- Once we know who we are more likely to 'clash' with, we can try and blend in a bit better (self-management) to avoid conflict.

- If we do end up in conflict we will behave in an assertive way (this is completely different from aggressive although the terms are often misused) and aim to find a win–win situation.

- A good leader will be able to switch to using four different leaderships styles when appropriate and will avoid micro-management or pacesetting. (This pacesetting style currently dominates the NHS in both clinical and non-clinical leaders.)

- Remember when giving feedback and praise:

  - Situation Behaviour Impact Change or Continue

- Knowing where everything is and having it laid out in a logical, clearly marked way not only makes it more efficient but it makes it safer

- Standardizing the layout of clinical areas decreases errors

- If you are doing a transfer, plan and plan some more.

- Try not to interrupt others. If you are interrupted yourself, start the task again if you can and watch for errors.

- Try not to stand over patients in their beds and talk down to them. Always imagine how they might be feeling.

- SBAR—situation, background, assessment, recommendation/request— is good for handovers of information especially on the phone.

- 'Active identification' needs to become standard practice with all drug administration and before any procedure and before any clinical interaction.

- It is possible to design equipment to eliminate layers of cheese and to decrease the chance of error.

- Being adequately trained on a piece of equipment is essential. Subsequent skill maintenance is also essential, particularly if the kit is used infrequently.

- Training with simulation offers an alternative for acquiring and maintaining skills.

- If your physiological needs are not being met leaving you hungry, thirsty, tired, or in need of the toilet, you are more likely to make a mistake.

- The 'two breath' technique can help manage your stress levels in a crisis. An alternative is the 'in for 7 out 11' approach.

- We will all suffer life events at some point, be careful how these can impact on you at work.

- We have stressful jobs. Don't be afraid to ask for support. Those around you will need support too.

- Each shift should start with a brief to highlight where that day's errors might crop up and to try to achieve a share mental model from the outset.

- Each shift should finish with a debrief. A debrief is a learning conversation that reinforces positive parts of the day and highlights changes as a result of errors or nearly events.

- A debrief is also required after a crisis situation where it also serves the purpose of supporting the staff involved.

- A large part of transfer of information (communication) is non-verbal. This means that mis-communication is more likely by phone or text or email or in patients' notes or letters.

- Starting with the big picture and then 'funnelling' down to the detail is a useful framework for information transfer.

8

Error awareness

If you don't make mistakes, you don't make anything

Late nineteenth-century proverb

Introduction

There is a school of thought that if we practise looking for errors, just like we practise many other skills in healthcare, then we will improve at it. If we can start identifying potential errors before they happen, we have time to change what is happening and hopefully avert the error. The aim of this final chapter is to do some of that practice. I would like to give you a series of examples. I would like you to analyse the story using the SHEEP sheet and spot errors. We will then consider what steps we could put in to avert the error. We will be emphasizing again that the Reason model of the Swiss cheese holes is important. There is not one causal factor, so there is not one single step to make it safer. We need to get better at looking at multiple factors and how they interact. At the end of the chapter we talk about using the learning from a near miss or 'nearly' event rather than always waiting until something serious has happened. In other words we want to move away from a stable door, horse already bolted scenario to one when we realize that the horse might be about to run out but we manage to stop it.

It works much better if you can find a piece of paper at this point. I realize for some this will go against the grain. Please write down the contributory factors as we progress through each example (see Examples 8.1–8.10).

Examples section—Swiss cheese practice

Example 8.1

The new doctor (foundation trainee) arrived on the ward on their second week to be met with a frown from the ward clerk. The ward round had started early but the junior doctor hadn't received the email from the Consultant's secretary to inform them of the change of time. The Consultant scowled at the doctor as they arrived (late). The junior doctor has missed visiting the first two patients (in beds 3 and 5). The junior stared at the floor and apologized. The nursing staff are struggling this morning as someone is off sick. There are not enough nurses for someone to come on the ward round. You could cut the atmosphere with a knife and the junior (Dr Brown) is a high flyer who likes to be a perfectionist. Dr Brown is desperate to please and attempts to make a good impression for the rest of the ward round. The more senior members of the team go straight to theatre after the end of the ward round leaving Dr Brown to manage the wards. Dr Brown works very hard after the ward round and misses lunch, determined to try and make up for earlier. Dr Brown stays late to finish everything that needed doing but continues to worry about the impression they made today. The next day, Dr Brown arrives early and goes to visit Mrs Rose in bed 3. Mrs Rose's bed is surrounded by lots of people: several nurses, the Outreach team, and someone from ICU. Mrs Rose appears to have become septic. Dr Brown's registrar asks why the blood gas wasn't done yesterday and why the antibiotics hadn't been started as the Consultant had requested. Dr Brown said they knew nothing about those requests. A very aggressive conversation ensues at the end of the bed with the Registrar blaming Dr Brown.

No one intervenes. Dr Brown explains that they had followed the instructions in the notes but there was no mention of blood gas or antibiotics. The registrar snatches the notes. The CT1 or SHO (next level of doctor up from foundation training) had written the notes until Dr Brown had arrived. The Consultant never allowed much time for documentation on their ward rounds. The notes were very scanty and not very legible. There is no mention of a blood gas or antibiotics in the notes. The CT1 arrives and the Registrar asks them about writing it down or doing a handover. The CT1 claims that they told Dr Brown.

Dr Brown bursts into tears just as Mr Rose arrives on the ward with his son and daughter.

I hope you would be as concerned as me that Mrs Rose has had her safety compromised and that the experience for her and also for her relatives has been less than ideal. This standard of care is not something we would be proud of. This care would not be what we wanted for ourselves or for our families.

I would like you to count how many factors you think may have contributed to this problem for Mrs Rose. If you are not yet convinced about the worth of writing it down, then please feel free to do it all in your head. However, I hope that you might make the time to use the SHEEP sheet as we have already considered the benefits of cognitive aids.

For each tick, I would like you to consider if there is a solution or change that could be implemented to eliminate, or at least decrease the likelihood of, that slice of cheese lining up.

1. Dr Brown is new to the job. You are more likely to make a mistake early in a new job. Whilst we cannot stop people being new, we can ensure that they are adequately inducted. This involves familiarization with systems, staff, environments, team preferences, equipment, and the organization. In this case, knowing that the Consultant has a tendency to alter the time of the ward round on the day they run a theatre list would have been useful information.

2. Email is not a true form of communication (information transfer) as it fails to fulfil some of the steps. It falsely gives the idea that information has been delivered. Face to face is best. If it has to be by phone, text, or email, remember that 'read back' is necessary to confirm receipt of the message and clarification of understanding. If the Consultant had told Dr Brown to their face that the ward round would be starting early and checked for transfer of information, Dr Brown would not have been late.

3–5. The ward clerk, the Consultant, and the team as a whole were not welcoming or inclusive. Good team working has been shown to have a positive effect on mortality.

6. There was no handover of information about the early patients in the ward round. Let alone a handover using a standardized format like SBAR which improves information transfer.

7–9. The ward round technique did not allow adequate time for documentation. The documentation of the requests for blood gas and antibiotics was not documented. What was documented was scanty and was also illegible.

10–11. There is no summary phase of the ward round to generate a job list or to help with prioritization of tasks. Instead the senior members of the team leave to go to another clinical area and do not return or check that the team are coping.

12. There are cultural issues that the most junior members of the team are left to cope in some instances without adequate levels of supervision.

13–14. Blood gases were not done. Antibiotics were not prescribed. Whilst the CT1 claims that they gave Dr Brown a verbal handover of the tasks, as above an SBAR-style handover and documentation of a task list would be better.

15. Nursing sickness meant that there were no nurses present on the ward round, whilst this may usually have served to be a double check that tasks were carried out. There was no handover to the nursing staff at the end of each bay or even each ward.

16. There was certainly not a learning debrief that was supportive and encouraged an open culture. None of the 15 learning points listed were captured and acted upon so that they wouldn't happen again . . .

There were more issues but I hope this list illustrates the idea of the multiple layers of cheese contributing to the errors.

Example 8.2

There is a busy obstetric clinic. Mrs Smith is waiting to be seen in room 2. Mrs Jones is shown into room 4. The consultant and the associate specialist and the senior house officer/CT2 are all involved in trying to get through the clinic which is heavily overbooked. The usual nurse who runs the outpatient clinic is on annual leave. The person standing in is more senior than the usual one and knows the area well. Each patient has their urine dipped and their observations (blood pressure) taken before they are seen. There are six different clinic rooms. As the associate specialist emerges from room 3, they look concerned. Mrs Fothergill in room 5 has not felt her baby moving since yesterday. The associate specialist waits for the consultant to emerge from room 1. As the consultant walks out the efficient nurse hands them the notes for Mrs Smith in room 2. 'Mrs Smith, room 2, twins'. The associate specialist and the CT2 approach the consultant from either side and both give a brief handover of their cases. The consultant suggests advice to the CT2 for Mrs Paul in room 4 and takes the notes for Mrs Fothergill. The consultant's pager then goes off. They answer the pager with both sets of notes tucked under their arm. A complex conversation ensues about the bed state on labour ward and whether there will be safe staffing levels for the afternoon shift. There is quite a balance of political pressure and emotion within the conversation. The consultant can finally return to the clinic. The consultant heads off to room 2. 'Mrs . . . ' hesitates the consultant. Glances at the notes and sees the name on the front, 'Smith?'

'Yes.'

'I think in view of what I've been told we need an urgent ultrasound to check everything is OK. I will just fill in this form. Do you know where the scan room is?' They confirm the directions between them. Mrs Smith heads off for a scan looking worried.

> As the consultant comes out of the room, the nurse gives them another set of notes, 'Mrs Jones, room 4, pre-eclampsia last pregnancy, BP 125/65 today'.
>
> The associate specialist asks, 'How is she?'.
>
> 'I've sent her for an urgent scan', replies the consultant.
>
> 'I'm one behind, I need to see the twins lady next . . . '.

At this point we have a mother of twins terrified that she has a problem when none is known and a mother who may have a problem still sitting in a room unseen. Let's stop it there.

I would like you to take the time again to either use the SHEEP sheet as a prompt or to scribble a list of contributory factors and a solution for each where possible.

1. High workload makes an error more likely—the clinic was overbooked.

2. Member of regular staff on leave. Usual systems may not be followed.

3. Multiple patients in multiple rooms creates an environment where ambiguity and risk of misidentification are possible.

4. Interruptions disturb cognitive processes and often contribute to error. The emotional, political, and financial pressures of the conversation mean that it will be very distracting.

5. Use of pronouns (she) rather than confirmation of the patient's name allows the ambiguity to persist longer.

6. Lack of 'active identification' allows a wrong patient wrong information moment.

7. Lack of 'read back' means room and patient information is not double checked.

Example 8.3

Mr Cotes had suffered a stroke 10 days previously. It had been complicated and he required ventilation on intensive care. He had a tracheostomy inserted and was now recovering on a ward. He was being cared for on the respiratory ward as in this hospital they were fully trained in tracheostomy management. He required regular chest physiotherapy and regular suction by the ward staff, in addition to his post-stroke care. He was making slow progress but progress none the less. The hospital was filled over capacity. The person responsible for bed management at night needed to fill a bed on a surgical outlying ward to free up a space on the respiratory ward. There was no one available to take the phone call when the bed manager phoned the ward, the phone just rang and rang. It was 10.30pm. The respiratory patient in the emergency department was about to breech the 4-hour wait time. The bed manager went to the ward but was unable to speak to the nurse in charge who was helping with an acute asthmatic. She spoke to the only other qualified nurse on the ward at that moment who hurriedly glanced down her handover list and suggested Mr Cotes—he had had a stroke and wasn't even a respiratory patient anyway. The porters arrived shortly after and Mr Cotes was transferred to the surgical ward. The family were not informed of the move. The move was not cleared with the nurse-in-charge. Mr Cotes was moved three more times over the next 3 days to three different wards.

That night his tracheostomy became displaced. The ward staff had little experience with tracheostomies. It was dark. Mr Cotes was not near the nurses' station. No one noticed initially. When he was found he was peri-arrest. A crash call went out and by the time the team arrived he was in full cardiac arrest. Despite a successful return of circulation, Mr Cotes suffered hypoxic brain damage.

Unfortunately, this one is not make-believe but was told to me by a friend about their relative. The name has, of course, been changed.

How would you feel if you found out this happened in your hospital?
Can you spot all the layers of cheese?
What solutions might you employ to try and make things safer?

Example 8.4

Mrs Rose from Example 8.1 never made it out of intensive care, she died after 13 days.

Mr Rose wishes to make a complaint. He has spent time with the patient liaison service and some of the intensive care team but it is the ward team with whom he is angry. He just wants to know what happened. The Medical

Director has reviewed the notes and found them to be rather illegible and scanty at best. He is talking to the family today with one of the Matrons.

One of the administrators has arranged for the Matron to meet the family at the entrance with one of the patient liaison team. Mr Rose is bringing his son and daughter for support.

Rose family	Matron
'I can't believe they are not here waiting to meet us after all we have been through!' 'Where are they?' Looks at his letter. 'Main entrance. 11am.' 'Well here we are!'	'I'm glad I'm early, I feel that we have put them through enough.' 'They were very punctual when I saw them previously.' 'I'll just phone Brenda and check I've got the time right.' 'Brenda? The Rose family aren't here yet. Can you just check the letter for me?' 'Main entrance. 11am.'
'I'm getting a bit fed up with this!' Mr Rose's son takes out his mobile and phones the number on the letter. 'We are supposed to have someone meeting us! My father is elderly! You have already killed my mother!' 'What do you mean there is someone here waiting—do you think I am stupid? We are at the entrance now! Yes, by the car park! No, there is not a statue in the foyer! No, there is not a coffee shop in front of me either! It might have been helpful to explain that there are two foyers before we came!'	'Brenda, I'm sorry to bother you, but they are still not here. Have you got their contact details handy?'

I think it would be fair to assume that an already difficult meeting about the circumstances surrounding Mrs Rose's death will now be even more challenging. There are two main entrances to this particular hospital. Both are close to a car park. The conversation previously had involved some attempt at confirming understanding. The administrator had asked, 'Do you know where that is?' and of course, Mr Rose was unaware that there were two options. He assumed that his mental model was the correct one. He did not know that in Brenda's mind she was picturing the one with the statue and the coffee shop. Brenda had a different mental model.

Mr Rose could not have known there were two car parks and two entrances; it was an 'unknown unknown'.

Brenda had tried hard to communicate with Mr Rose. She had sent a letter and made a phone call to confirm the appointment. Brenda did not use a funnelling system that started with the big picture and then progress to the detail. There was no 'read back' used to check for a shared mental model and no full confirmation of information transfer. There was no map of the hospital with an 'X' marks the spot. There was no consideration of the possible ambiguity of the two car parks and the two entrances by the other members of staff either. It is easy to be accepting of information that you are given, especially from someone who is usually completely reliable and trusted. We always need to ask ourselves the right questions. Is there anything missing here?

Brenda, the Matron, the patient liaison team, and the Medical Director may all learn from this error and not make the same mistake themselves again. The real question is, how will others learn from it?

What is the mechanism for organizational learning where you work?

Example 8.5

Standing at the nurses' station the Registrar in paediatrics who is well liked and held in the highest regard is writing a drug prescription for the child in bed 5. She has identified the child, checked the weight against her estimate for age, and checked the name on the drug chart matches the notes. It is a simple prescription for paracetamol and diclofenac (pain killers). She has written the paracetamol dose first and is now writing the one for diclofenac when her bleep goes off. She deals with the phone call offering some advice to the more junior doctor on another ward. A nurse then comes to ask for advice on another patient.

She goes back to finishing her prescription for diclofenac and asks the nurse to dispense the medication politely and in good humour.

The nurse checks the prescription in the children's dosing guidelines (BNF). She notices that it is a high dose of diclofenac but assumes that Dr Ramsay is so reliable that must have been her intention. She gives the drug.

The alarm is raised shortly afterwards when another doctor is reviewing the child for another medical condition. The poisons unit is contacted for advice and management suggestions followed. A full discussion is had by the registrar about the error with both the patient and the mother.

No harm comes to the child . . . this time. And lessons are learnt.

Both Dr Ramsay and the nurse involved are very upset.

Example 8.6

A new drug chart is introduced to a hospital. Whilst there have been pilots in some areas to practise with the new chart not everyone has had training or even seen the new chart when it is introduced. Each ward spends the first part of handover discussing the new layout of the drug chart. They are warned to look for drug errors. Inevitably some staff are on leave when the transition phase occurs. It is a hot topic for a week or so and then the hyper-vigilance slips back to normal levels of 'comfort'.

A patient with a high BMI (body mass index) and diabetes has undergone major surgery. They are considered to be high risk for developing a postoperative deep vein thrombosis (DVT) or even a pulmonary embolus (PE). They have had some blood-thinning medicine prescribed. The prescription is on a separate page on the new chart. The drug is omitted for 3 days. Three shifts a day for 3 days.

On day 5 the patient develops a life-threatening PE.

Once a drug error involving an omission has taken place, it is likely that this will persist. There seems to be an assumption subconsciously that the omission must have been for a reason and so a further omission occurs. Once a series of omissions have occurred it is less and less likely to be spotted.

Example 8.7

There is an acute airway emergency in theatre 5 anaesthetic room. This is a 'Can't intubate, can't ventilate!'.

'Get the emergency airway trolley! It is outside theatre 4 in the corridor.'

ODP replies, 'Airway trolley, outside theatre 4—getting it now!'

'Cannula inserted, able to aspirate air . . . Pass me the end of the Sander's injector.'

'What do you mean there isn't one!? It must be there, in the box, look again!'

'Hold this – I'll look! Oh . . . 'expletive'!'

On this occasion, Example 8.7 had involved taking a manikin to theatre 5 anaesthetic room, but it had not been a set-up that part of the equipment was missing: that bit was horribly real. There was an audible sigh of relief that we had discovered the missing equipment in a simulated scenario rather than a real one. The lessons were learnt rather rapidly and the procedures for checking the emergency airway trolley were altered.

Example 8.8

As the senior resuscitation officer (I shall use the abbreviation resus officer) arrives at the bedside following an arrest call, there are already ten staff crammed around the bed. She stands back briefly to try and take stock of the situation. It is not obvious who is leading. In fact, it is not obvious what roles most people have. There is certainly someone taking the airway, another two trying to get intravenous access (one on each arm), chest compressions are happening (although how effective they are might be debateable), and someone is attaching the defibrillator pads. She notices it is one of the able but less confident senior house officers (CT2) who should be leading things but they seem to be having a 'bunny in the headlights moment'. She has to make a quick decision: to take over and risk undermining confidence further or to try and coach her through it. She opts for the latter.

'Who's leading?' asks the resus officer.

'I am!' replies the CT2. This seems to be enough to have intervened with the bunny moment.

The resus officer uses non-verbal communication to subtly encourage the CT2 to stand at the end of bed. She quietly encourages and asks poignant questions about the rhythm, the side of the algorithm we are on (shockable or non-shockable), how roles might need to be allocated, and the way all of this might need to be communicated with the team.

Before long the oxygen is attached to the Ambu bag and so we are no longer giving room air which is only 21% oxygen, the compressions are adequate, someone is allocated to giving the drugs, all of those without a clear role are waiting for instructions at the end of bed, someone is collecting the notes and reading out relevant information, someone is time keeping and writing notes, and the atmosphere of chaos has been replaced by order and logic. The CT2 has found their stride and the arrest is running as smoothly as they ever do.

Unfortunately, as with a large number of non-shockable arrests this one is not successful. The medical registrar arrives and an excellent handover of the situation is given in an SBAR framework backed up by the notes of the arrest which have been recorded real time. There is a full team discussion but eventually the decision has to be made that despite every effort, they will not be successful on this occasion. The time of death is called.

The resus officer takes the team aside for a debrief. Everyone is given a chance to say how they feel it went and offer up any learning that they might take away. There is an opportunity to emphasize the need for giving the oxygen and not falling into the trap of giving only room air. The need for compressions to be deep enough and fast enough is also discussed. The team praise the CT2 who goes away with renewed self-belief. The team are able to express their sadness and disappointment at the outcome. They are reassured that they did everything that they could. Ongoing support is offered if any of them need it.

The resus officer goes away happy knowing that they managed to keep the patient's interests first and foremost but managed to achieve this without taking over: a challenging balance but worth achieving.

Example 8.9

An intensive care unit was full. There was another patient who needed intensive care. There were no patients who were ready for discharge and all other options for the care of this patient had been exhausted. There was no choice but to transfer the patient to another intensive care unit. The transfer was uneventful and the patient made good progress and was ready for a ward bed a few days later.

The receiving hospital phoned the medical registrar at the transferring hospital. The medical registrar took the attitude that it was not their problem and was not cooperative and, in fact, was not even polite.

The receiving hospital contacted the intensive care consultant at the base hospital. The consultant was very apologetic on behalf of the medical registrar and promised to help find a solution. The receiving consultant explained that they needed to admit another patient to their unit.

The consultant intensivist did not want to burn any bridges, they relied on the cooperation between the two units and they needed it to work well.

The consultant intensivist called the physician consultant who was on call who was very helpful. Despite being full the two consultants managed to find a solution to take the patient back. This involved the consultant intensivist being on the phone for around 45 minutes.

Is this the best use of consultant time?

During this time, the consultant had missed part of the ward round. A post-operative patient who had been on intensive care for 2 days after a complicated operation had a good epidural in place which was providing them with good pain relief and was allowing the patient to cough well and cooperate with their physiotherapy. The consultant wanted them to return to the ward with the epidural still running. They did not get chance to offer up this information as the patient had been discharged while they were on the phone. This did not come to light until 2 days later when the same consultant was called to review the patient in view of the deterioration in respiratory function on the ward.

On questioning the patient, once the epidural had been stopped, they said they found coughing and the deep breathing exercises too painful. The patient had stopped doing both as they were inadequately analgesed.

Neither consultant explained to the medical registrar about the consequence of their actions. No one dealt with the attitude or behaviour which was less than professional. The medical registrar remained unaware of the potential impact they might have had on future intensive care transfers and no learning took place. On intensive care there was a 'debrief' session to discuss the re-admission of the patient. There was a brief teaching session on the importance of postoperative pain relief and a discussion about communication at the time of discharge. There was a brief brainstorm about following up patients who have been discharged more closely. There were lots of learning points identified and people came up with their own ideas about how to make systems better. There was no blame or finger pointing. It was a safe, productive debrief. When asked if people had found it helpful, the responses were very positive. When asked if they would like to do it again, there was a resounding 'yes'.

A man who reviews the old so as to find out the new is qualified to teach others.

Confucius (551–479 BC), *Analects*, Chapter 2, Verse 11.

Example 8.10

The consultant anaesthetist had taken a thorough preoperative assessment and had explained everything to the patient prior to their surgery for incision and drainage of an abscess. The patient was starved and completely fit and healthy with a normal preoperative blood sugar. They were a non-smoker with no known allergies and had previously had an uneventful general anaesthetic. They had no reflux and normal dentition. The airway assessment was compatible with the findings of a previously easy intubation. All ward checks had been completed by both the ward staff and the surgical team. The WHO checklist was carried out thoroughly at each stage. All drugs and equipment were checked. All staff were appropriately trained. Everyone had had enough sleep, enough breaks, and no major life events. There was no high work load that day. The patient had no unexpected anatomy or physiology and everything went smoothly.

There were no errors.

We need to aim not only to capture learning from when an error has occurred but to move to the next step to prevent them.

By starting to capture learning from nearly events (near misses) we may be able to put in place some of the interventions before it is too late, before we have to meet relatives and talk about how we failed their loved one.

We may be able to prevent deaths like those of Elaine Bromiley and Beth Bowen and my friend Carol and my dad, from happening.

I hope you will join with me in an apology to all of those people and their families and the many like them from us, the healthcare staff.

We need to be open about our mistakes.

We need to learn from our mistakes.

I hope you will join with me in promising to change things: we need to make it better.

Key points from all chapters

- ◆ To err is human.
- ◆ The commonest type of mistake is poor communication but we are going to think of this as a failure of information transfer.
- ◆ By using 'read back' and clarification we can increase the chances of successful information transfer.
- ◆ We all make mistakes. We can get better at anticipating them with practice. Are you looking at how to avoid your next one?

- We need to embed an open culture. What might your first steps be to help this become a reality?

- There should be an inquisitive approach to error that seeks out the learning and shares it: the learning culture.

- How is learning shared in your organization?

- The new error checklist—the SHEEP sheet—helps gather more information following an actual event or a nearly event. The SHEEP sheet can be used for trend analysis. By looking at trends, preventative measures can be targeted.

- Information flow across an organization can be achieved using a brief/debrief model using Debbie's Diamond.

- Systems errors are commonly part of the holes in the Swiss cheese and should feature in the solutions for improved safety.

- It is really hard to avoid assumptions. What methods are you going to employ?

- 'What am I missing here?' is a healthy question to keep asking.

- If the hierarchy is too steep, the team will not feel able to challenge the leader if they are making a mistake.

- We all make mistakes.

- If there is a flat hierarchy and no natural leader emerges, ask the question, 'Who's leading?'.

- Followership is a much overlooked and important skill to have. One aspect is being assertive enough to speak up if things are about to go wrong.

- We will all push someone else's buttons. We can't change the other person, only ourselves.

- We need to become more aware of how we are impacting on others (increase our self-awareness). This might begin with knowing our preferred learning style, team role, and our personality type (MBTI).

- Once we know who we are more likely to 'clash' with, we can try and blend in a bit better (self-management) to avoid conflict.

- If we do end up in conflict we will behave in an assertive way (this is completely different from aggressive although the terms are often misused) and aim to find a win–win situation.

- A good leader will be able to switch to using four different leaderships styles when appropriate and will avoid micro-management or pacesetting. (This pacesetting style currently dominates the NHS in both clinical and non-clinical leaders.)

- Remember when giving feedback and praise:

  - Situation Behaviour Impact Change or Continue

- Knowing where everything is and having it laid out in a logical, clearly marked way not only makes it more efficient but it makes it safer.

- Standardizing the layout of clinical areas decreases errors.

- If you are doing a transfer, plan and plan some more.

- Try not to interrupt others. If you are interrupted yourself, start the task again if you can and watch for errors.

- Try not to stand over patients in their beds and talk down to them. Always imagine how they might be feeling.

- SBAR—situation, background, assessment, recommendation/request— is good for handovers of information, especially on the phone.

- 'Active identification' needs to become standard practice with all drug administration and before any procedure and before any clinical interaction.

- It is possible to design equipment to eliminate layers of cheese and to decrease the chance of error.

- Being adequately trained on a piece of equipment is essential. Subsequent skill maintenance is also essential, particularly if the kit is used infrequently.

- Training with simulation offers an alternative for acquiring and maintaining skills.

- If your physiological needs are not being met leaving you hungry, thirsty, tired, or in need of the toilet, you are more likely to make a mistake.

- The 'two-breath' technique can help manage your stress levels in a crisis. An alternative is the 'in for 7 out 11' approach.

- We will all suffer life events at some point, be careful how these can impact on you at work.

- We have stressful jobs. Don't be afraid to ask for support. Those around you will need support too.

- Each shift should start with a brief to highlight where that day's errors might crop up and to try to achieve a share mental model from the outset.

- Each shift should finish with a debrief. A debrief is a learning conversation that reinforces positive parts of the day and highlights changes as a result of errors or nearly events.

- A debrief is also required after a crisis situation where it also serves the purpose of supporting the staff involved.

- A large part of transfer of information (communication) is non-verbal. This means that miscommunication is more likely by phone, text, or email, or in patients' notes or letters.

- Starting with the big picture and then 'funnelling' down to the detail is a useful framework for information transfer.

- Listening is not the same as waiting to speak!

- Positivity is a great attribute of a team member.

- Don't be a mood-hoover!

- Praise people.

A final thought

Knowledge is proud that he has learned so much;

Wisdom is humble that he knows no more.

William Cowper (1731–1800), *The Task* (1785), Book 6, 'The Winter Walk at Noon', Line 96.

The SHEEP sheet (Figure A.1)

Systems

CULTURE

HOSPITAL CULTURE
- [ ] Departmental
- [ ] Professional
- [ ] Workgroup
- [ ] Mgmt vs. clinical
- [ ] Leadership culture

CULTURAL SYSTEMS LACK OF
- [ ] Open culture
- [ ] Safety culture
- [ ] Reporting Culture

INFORMATION FLOW CHOICE OF
- [ ] Face to face
- [ ] Phone
- [ ] Email
- [ ] Text
- [ ] Fax
- [ ] Access to info systems
- [ ] Access to info sets
- [ ] Briefing
- [ ] Debriefing
- [ ] Handover

INFORMATION SYSTEMS

MANUAL
- [ ] Patient notes
- [ ] Clinical pathway
- [ ] Care bundles

AUTOMATED APPLICATION
- [ ] Theatre mgmt
- [ ] Bed mgmt
- [ ] Pathology
- [ ] Patient mgmt

INFRASTRUCTURE
- [ ] Network
- [ ] Hardware

PRESCRIBED (SOP/Protocol/Guideline Issue)

- [ ] Failure to follow
  - [ ] National
  - [ ] Local
  - [ ] Legal & Binding
  - [ ] WHO checklist
  - [ ] Care Bundle
  - [ ] Research
  - [ ] Professional Body
- [ ] Lack of familiarity
- [ ] Different versions
- [ ] Ambiguity within
- [ ] Ambiguity between
- [ ] Unable to locate
- [ ] Chose to deviate due to
  - [ ] Experience
  - [ ] Out of date
  - [ ] Inappropriate to situation
- [ ] Refusal to use
- [ ] Complexity
- [ ] Not understood
- [ ] Conflicting rules/ guidelines

IMPROVEMENT MODELS

LACK OF
- [ ] Productive ward
- [ ] TPOT (the productive operating theatre)
- [ ] Lean/6Sigma

ORGANIZATIONAL FLOW

PROBLEM WITH
- [ ] Clinical Department
- [ ] Business Department
- [ ] HR Department
- [ ] Finance Department
- [ ] IT Department
- [ ] Estates Department
- [ ] Quality Control
- [ ] Infection Control
- [ ] Security Systems

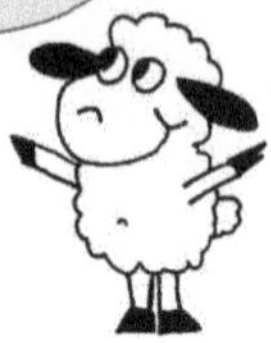

Equipment

GENERIC PROBLEM WITH EQUIPMENT ITSELF

- [ ] Fitness for task
- [ ] Manufacturing
- [ ] Supply
- [ ] Storage
- [ ] Availability
  - [ ] Location
  - [ ] In stock
  - [ ] Timely access
- [ ] Readiness for use
  - [ ] Cleanliness
  - [ ] Working order
  - [ ] Maintained
- [ ] Accuracy
- [ ] Reliability
- [ ] Safety
- [ ] Equipment Compatibility
  - [ ] Electrical
- [ ] Safety coding
  - [ ] Colour
  - [ ] Device interconnection
- [ ] Model of equipment
- [ ] Equipment Failure

DRUGS
- [ ] Prescribing abbreviated
- [ ] Prescribing illegible
- [ ] Prescribing wrong drug
- [ ] Prescribing wrong dose
- [ ] Prescribing wrong frequency
- [ ] Interactions between drugs
- [ ] Duplication
- [ ] Multiple charts
- [ ] Ambiguity
  - [ ] Dispensing
  - [ ] Preparation
  - [ ] Administer
- [ ] Wrong patient
- [ ] Wrong drug
- [ ] Wrong route
- [ ] Time delay
- [ ] Frequency
  - [ ] Too frequent
  - [ ] Too infrequent
- [ ] Wrong dose
- [ ] Wrong equipment
- [ ] Wrong technique

CONSUMABLES
- [ ] Sterility
- [ ] Shelf life
- [ ] Administer
  - [ ] Wrong patient
  - [ ] Wrong consumable
  - [ ] Incompatible
  - [ ] Left in patient

NON CONSUMABLES
- [ ] Bed design
- [ ] Bed mechanical failure
- [ ] Bed electrical failure
- [ ] Bed mattress problem
- [ ] Bedrails
- [ ] Shower curtains
- [ ] Other

Personal

EXTERNAL INFLUENCES

PROBLEMS WITH
- [ ] Mood
- [ ] Frustration
- [ ] Emotional security
- [ ] Emotional trigger (events)
- [ ] Feeling unprepared
- [ ] Failure to achieve expectations
- [ ] Lack of self awareness
- [ ] Confidence
- [ ] Self esteem
- [ ] Motivation
- [ ] Lack of interest
- [ ] Complacency
- [ ] Denial of the situation
- [ ] Adaptability
- [ ] Ability to cope with major change
- [ ] Ability to cope with interruptions

PROBLEMS INFLUENCED BY WHO YOU ARE
- [ ] Race
- [ ] Gender
- [ ] Sexuality
- [ ] Personal value systems
- [ ] Personality (MBTI)
- [ ] Morals
- [ ] Cultural Identity

PATHOLOGY/PHYSIOLOGY
- [ ] Tired
- [ ] Hungry
- [ ] Thirsty
- [ ] Toilet break
- [ ] Health/illness
  - [ ] Untreated (or)
  - [ ] On treatment
- [ ] Stressed
- [ ] No energy
- [ ] Hormones/pregnancy

LIFE EVENTS
- [ ] Children
- [ ] Family
- [ ] Relationships
- [ ] Divorce
- [ ] Bereavement
- [ ] House move
- [ ] An argument
- [ ] Friends
- [ ] Commuting
- [ ] Parking
- [ ] Addiction to drugs
- [ ] Addiction to alcohol

ATTITUDES, BEHAVIOUR & EMOTION

MY WORK PROBLEMS WITH
- [ ] An argument
- [ ] Poor morale
- [ ] Time pressure
- [ ] Lack of planning time
- [ ] Work time
- [ ] Rest time
- [ ] Work/rest balance
- [ ] Time of day
- [ ] Shift pattern
- [ ] Task conditions
  - [ ] Elective
  - [ ] Scheduled
  - [ ] Urgent
  - [ ] Emergency
  - [ ] Clinical
  - [ ] Non clinical
- [ ] High workload
- [ ] Lack of job satisfaction
- [ ] Job security
- [ ] Lack of team fit
- [ ] Lack of sense of belonging

Figure A.1 The SHEEP sheet.

Human Interaction

TEAM DYNAMICS & CONFLICT

PROBLEMS WITH TEAM
- Personality types
- Unclear team roles
- Preferred team role
- Perceived unfairness
- Perceived vs actual power
- Accountability
- Approach to change
- Difference in preferred communication styles
- Difference in preferred learning styles
- Mixed messages
- Preconceived ideas
- Conflicting expectations
- Skill mix

PROBLEMS WITH
- Patient interaction
- Conflict visibility
  - Observable
  - Hidden

PROBLEMS WITH LEADER
- Leadership styles
- Lack of leadership
- Lack of followership
- Hierarchy too steep
- Hierarchy too flat

BEHAVIOURS

INTERACTION QUALITY
- Challenging (negative) behaviour
- Lack of diversity consideration (gender, sex, culture, age)
- Prejudice
- Aggression
- Laziness
- Rudeness
- Snobbery
- Dishonesty
- Lack of consideration
- Lack of respect
  - of others
  - by others

- Over familiarity
- Empire building
- Trying to impress
- Negative responses
- Loss of sense of humour
- Unwillingness
- Apathy
- Fear
- Insecurity
- Making assumptions
- Reluctance to change
- Malicious intent

PROBLEMS WITH COMMUNICATION QUALITY
- Encoding
- Delivery
- Receipt
- Decoding
- Clarification
- Duplication
- Ambiguity
- Listening ability (receiving)
- Body language (non verbal)

Environment

LOCATION CHANGE

PROBLEMS WITH USER INTERACTION WITH EQUIPMENT
- Knowledge/Skill
  - Training
  - Experience
  - Frequency of use
  - Familiarity
  - Ability to troubleshoot
- Personal preference for equipment
- Availability of back-up equipment
- Ergonomic design/layout
  - User Interface
  - Ease of Use
  - Complexity
  - Readability
- Processing information
- Acting on information
- Post procedures check

INSTRUMENTS
- Sterility
- Administer
  - Wrong patient
  - Wrong instrument
  - Incompatible
  - Left in patient

MEDICAL GASES
- Prescribing
- Administer
  - Wrong patient
  - Wrong gas
  - Wrong delivery method
  - Wrong time
  - Wrong dose

HUMAN TISSUE, BLOOD PRODUCTS & TRANSPLANTATION
- Collection
- Processing
- Prescribing
- Preparation
  - Cross matching
  - Other preparation
- Administer
  - Wrong patient
  - Wrong blood/ Product/organ
  - Wrong route
  - Wrong time
    - Point
    - Delay
    - Duration
  - Wrong dose

- Patient monitor failure

IMPLANTS/PROSTHESES
- Functionality
- Insertion

PROBLEMS WITH JOURNEY BETWEEN LOCATIONS
- Complexity
- Distance
- Accessibility
  - Size
  - Secure areas
- Modality of transfer
  - Foot
  - Chair
  - Trolley/bed/stretcher
  - Vehicle
  - Lift/elevator
  - Lifting device (Hoist)

INTERRUPTIONS
- People
- Equipment, Bleep
- Phones
- Machines
- Media (text, email)

PHYSICAL PROBLEMS WITH
- Atmospheric composition (air)
- Temperature
- Humidity
- Smell
- Lighting
- Noise
- Cleanliness
- Size
- Security
- Tidiness

ERGONOMICS

PHYSICAL DESIGN PROBLEMS WITH
- Infrastructure (walls etc)
- Immovable structures (cupboards)
- Movable structures (beds, chairs)

TASK RELATED DESIGN PROBLEMS WITH
- Resource location
- Knowing where it is
- Visibility
- Accessible
- Organised
- Standardised
- Optimised

SAFETY CONTROLS
- Radiation
- Electromagnetic field (eg MRI, laser)
- Biochemical hazard

FUNCTIONAL DESIGN PROBLEMS WITH
- Proximity to eating/ resting/physiological function areas
- Privacy

VICINITY
- Arms reach area
- Immediate vicinity (no doors)
- Departmental area
- Hospital/GP practice/
- Clinical unit
- External

Generic Non–Technical Skills (G–NO–TECS) Debrief Prompt (Table A.1)

Generic Non-Technical Skills (G–NO–TECS) Debrief Prompt[1]	COMMENTS

Team
• Leadership skills (including approachability of leader)
• Followership skills (including assertiveness of followers)
• Team building and maintaining (including hierarchy management)
  ○ Clear and appropriate role allocation
  ○ Consideration and support of others
• Conflict solving	

Decision–Making • Problem definition and diagnosis (commentating, generating shared mental model) • Option generation (encouraging team input, avoiding fixation error) • Risk assessment and option selection • Regular review of decision as new information emerges	
Tasks • Providing and maintaining standards • Workload management (including distraction management and prioritization of tasks) • Knowledge of and ability to use equipment	
Awareness – Situational • Awareness of the systems • Awareness of the environment • Awareness of time (use of time checks) • Ability to plan ahead (anticipate need for staf f/equipment/change of environment) • Maintenance of care, compassion and dignity **Awareness – Self** • Stress, fatigue, cognitive workload, time pressure, call for help if appropriate • Balcony and dance floor[2], Swan	
Information Management • Gathering of information (from patient, relatives, team, other teams, records) • Sharing of information (including use of structured handover tool e.g. SBAR) • Use of cognitive aids (guidelines, BNF, internet) • Listening, non-verbal and verbal communication • Read back, active identif ication, cross check, open questions, avoidance of pronouns	

1. Source: data from Flin RH et al, Development of the NOTECHS (Non-Technical Skills) system for assessing pilots' CRM skills, *Journal of Human Performance in Extreme Environments*, Volume 3, pp. 95–117, Copyright © 2003.
2. Ronald A. Heiftze, Leadership without Easy Answers, Harvard University Press, Cambridge, USA, Copyright © 1994.

Index